Dancing
AS THE
Body
OF
CONSCIOUSNESS

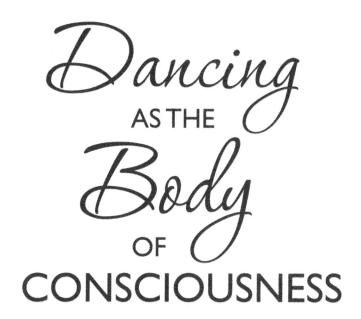

Dancing
AS THE
Body
OF
CONSCIOUSNESS

EDITOR
PATTY ALFONSO

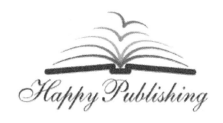

Happy Publishing

Secret bonuses just for you!

As a special thank you for buying our book, we'd like to invite you to be a part of our *Secret Bonuses Membership* page.

To access the site for free go to:

dancingasthebodyofconsciousness.com/secretbonuses

and enter your email address.

We are aware that this book is an invitation to a new way of being with your body. We have all been practicing these tools for many years and they have become part of us.

We would love to invite **you** to this new possibility.

We've created a place with additional resources, inspirational videos, quotes and much more so that you may begin your journey today.

These resources will guide you in having more joy, awareness, communion and fun with your body.

How much fun can you have with your body now?

Enjoy and thank you again for purchasing Dancing as the Body of Consciousness!

Acknowledgment

We would like to acknowledge the tools of Access Consciousness®.

These magical tools are both practical and pragmatic. If you are ready and willing, you can apply them to anything you are looking to change in your life and create the life and living you have always dreamed of.

A miraculous body of work, the tools include verbal processes as well as over 60 body processes to include your body on your journey towards consciousness.

For more information about these tools, and the amazing men who have spent decades sharing them with the world, you can go to:

www.AccessConsciousness.com
www.Body.AccessConsciousness.com
www.DrDainHeer.com
www.GaryMDouglas.com

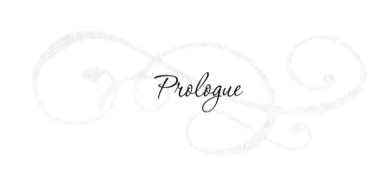

Prologue

I always knew I'd write a book. The energy of it has been present in my Universe for as long as I can remember. I just never knew when I would write or on what the subject would be.

In October 2015, after choosing to create more for my life and with my business, the urgency came rushing in as a whisper from the future: "The book, now..."

I still had no clue what I would be writing about and yet, I said: YES!

When I was at the Access Consciousness® 7-Day event in Costa Rica, I asked the Founder of Access Consciousness, Gary Douglas, if he would be willing to contribute a title for the book.

Curious, I watched him perceive the energy. Then he looked at me and said: *Dancing as the Body of Consciousness.* My whole body lit up and my universe expanded at the perception of the energy this title created in my body.

I then wondered: "What do other dancers, lovers of movement and bodies desire to say about dancing, the body and consciousness?" I tuned into the energy of the creation and asked: "Who? Show me please!"

And now, here we are...

Eight facilitators with eight different backgrounds sharing their journey with their bodies and the ways in which dance and movement contributes to creating a life greater than they can imagine.

I know each chapter will delight you energetically. The authors have all beautifully intertwined their stories with the tools from a space of being rather than explaining. A peak into a future possibility for you and your body. Enjoy the ride!

There is one tool I'd like to give you a sneak peek into before you begin your journey with us. That is the life-changing tool of: *Asking Questions*.

What you'll notice throughout the book is the use of questions that contributed to creating beyond what our logical minds can imagine.

In this reality we are taught to think. We are taught to use logic for everything. There is just one problem with this way of being in the world. The mind can only create based on what it *already knows*. When we function from our minds, we can only create based on our past experiences.

When you ask a question, without looking for an answer, you create an energetic opening for something new to show up. Questions open the door to new possibilities and new choices that weren't available in your limited, logical mind.

Are you ready for a different reality with your body, dance and movement? Are you ready to go beyond what you've been taught to something totally new, expansive and joyful?

We are certainly ready to share this with you! May this creation be as fun for you to read as it was for us to create!

Patty Alfonso

Access Consciousness® Certified Facilitator
Creator Pole Dancing For Consciousness™
Creator The Essence of You™

Table of Contents

Chapter 1

I am not a dancer...I just love to dance!
By Patty Alfonso

I've spent the last couple of years traveling.

Planes, trains and automobiles to and from 17 different countries around the world. I've walked and explored the streets of Tokyo, Paris, Florence, Copenhagen, London, Johannesburg, Monaco and Dubai to name a few.

I've been traveling for fun, for business, for classes, for obligations and for the pleasure of living.

What I haven't been doing too much of is dancing.

On the weeks when I wasn't traveling I did my best to go to the gym. Cycling, Zumba, Kickboxing and Yoga. Occasionally, I made it to a silks class and a Pole Dancing fitness class. But still... no dancing.

I noticed that the effort and force it took to go to the gym and move my body according to what someone else had decided was not only 'not fun', but it didn't create any joy for my body.

None of the aforementioned forms of movement are wrong. I'm just aware that they don't work for me and for my body.

I'm not a dancer, mind you. At least not a professional dancer. Dancing is just what my body loves to do!

Do you have something in your life that you just love to do? Something that brings you and your body pure joy?

What do I mean by dancing?

I should clarify. It's not just any dancing that I love… it's the kind of dancing where I don't have to follow any kind of routine.

The kind of dancing where I can let go of my mind and allow my body to be and move the way *she* desires to move.

The kind of dancing that melts everything away and allows me to simply be present with the music. Where I allow the music to move my body and create what I sense is a beautiful communion between my body, my being and the music.

You may be wondering what the heck I'm talking about right now! Let me share with you a bit about myself and my journey with dancing.

A ballerina is born or… maybe not…

When I was younger, I remember dancing all the time. Dancing all around the house, at restaurants and in school. I loved to dance.

I wasn't very coordinated though. Put me in a dance class and I was a mess! I simply couldn't follow the teacher's verbal instructions.

Getting what they were saying cognitively was a challenge. I had to see the entire move before I could do it and even then, I didn't want to do what they were doing. I wanted to do my own thing. I know now that this is due to my autistic capacities.

I took ballet lessons when I was little. The most fun I had

with ballet was when I was at home twirling and pirouetting around the house on my own.

Apparently, I did a little too much twirling and my grades in school suffered so I was quickly removed from ballet class.

You see, the body was not such an important "thing" in my family. Our intellect was prioritized over everything. Getting good grades, being in school, going to college, getting a job, being independent and then getting married. You know the drill.

That was the track my sister and I were supposed to follow. And, being the good daughter I wanted to be, I followed it.

Mind you, I'm not a good rule follower so, as you can imagine, I was always in trouble. Grades were never good enough, my behavior was never good enough and my choices were always wrong.

While in middle school and high school I was also involved in the drama club. I loved being on stage. I loved everything about the theater. The lighting, the music, the make-up and costumes, the audience, the laughter, the tears and the applause.

A few of my friends in school were dancers. Being trained in ballet and jazz, they had the opportunity to act and dance on stage and on TV.

I remember longing to have that as well. I remember begging my Mom to put me back in dance classes, to take me to an agent for representation and to auditions.

She promised she would but never did. My focus was to be solely on getting good grades. Since schoolwork was not my favorite thing to do, I never had the grades that would grant me the privilege of dancing again.

I had a friend in high school who came from a family of dancers. Her mother and sister were ballerinas. They were petite. My friend wasn't as slim as they were and she struggled with her weight and the pressure of having a "ballerina's body."

I always wondered why she was so unhappy about dancing and why she kept choosing it. She was in so much judgment about her body as she compared herself to other dancers.

In hindsight, I do wonder what my Mom knew about the dance world that she did not want to expose me to.

The older I got, the less I danced. With no dance classes to attend, and the emphasis on good grades, I became disconnected from the joy of moving that my body had come into this world with.

I was shy and introverted. And yet, if music was playing, I came alive.

My parents were extremely over-protective and controlling. My sister and I didn't have much of a social life when we were younger. We were very limited in the extracurricular activities we could participate in.

Luckily, we were allowed to be a part of a dance show that was filmed at WAPA TV in Puerto Rico.

It was called "Party-Time" and it featured special guests as well as the local community dancing and having a good time.

My friends and I would go every weekend for filming and dance. I loved the show, the dancing and being on TV. Everything I desired from my younger years showing up in a totally unexpected way!

Once I graduated from high school it was off to college. The only dancing I did there was in bars at clubs. Occasionally, I would pop into a Go-Go cage for fun. I loved being watched when I danced.

My friends would often make fun of me. There was a groove I would get into where everything would disappear except me, my body and the music.

I could hear them in the background: "There she goes again!" I didn't care though. My body and I were happy.

Dancing was the only time when I was truly happy. When I was truly having the joy of embodiment... the joy of having a body.

You see, with the intense focus on grades and the total disregard for my body, dancing was the only way my body got to be free from the thoughts, feelings and emotions that I allowed to rule my life.

There's no surprise that I was involved with the dramatic arts. I used to say that acting saved my life. It was one of the only places where I could express the energies I was aware of without getting into trouble.

My family wasn't into expressing anything. They were more into suppressing any energy that wasn't the illusion of perfection.

We are all infinite beings with the ability to perceive, know, be, and receive everything. When there is a suppression of energy, the energy gets pushed down.

But energy is constantly in motion and, while it's getting pushed down on one end, it must move out another. I was usually that other end.

At the time, I did not have any of the tools I have now to be aware of this. I was a constant explosion of energy moving. No wonder they thought I was a little crazy!

Since I was always in trouble, I eventually learned to suppress the energies I was aware of as well. It was only through movement and dance that I was able to unlock these energies from my body.

College came and went. I partied, danced, made amazing friends and miraculously graduated on time. Per my parents demand I had a "degree to fall back on" in case my dreams of acting did not come true. They were totally functioning from the "starving artist" point of view.

After college, I made the demand for me and for my life. I had done what my parents wanted and now it was time for what I desired.

I enrolled in drama classes, took ballet lessons again and started creating the life I thought I had always desired.

I pursued a career as an actor for many years. I had a bit role on a soap opera, did many commercials, independent films and theater.

I got bored though. Endless auditions and rejections. When I booked the job, I grew bored on set having to do the same thing over and over again. And I was bored with the sitting around waiting.

I WANTED MORE...

I got sober when I was 31 and enrolled in energy healing school in Los Angeles, CA. This choice changed the trajectory of my life in a way I could have never imagined.

As part of our curriculum, we had to find a kind of movement for our bodies. Beyond learning about chakras, QiGong, energy work, anatomy, and therapeutic techniques, we were required to get in touch with our bodies through movement.

Being slightly different, I ended up choosing pole dancing as my movement class. I was aware they expected me to choose something like yoga but the days of choosing what others expected of me were long gone.

And, having tried different kinds of yoga in the past, I already knew my body didn't really enjoy it. I did have a sense of peace after each class but I found holding the poses incredibly boring and quite torturous.

I enjoyed Kundalini Yoga a bit more as there was movement, but my body was still uninspired.

POLE DANCING:
A NEW WAY OF BEING WITH MY BODY

During my time at energy healing school, I had become aware that there was an energy that I was refusing to be. An energy in my body that I wasn't allowing to flow. I couldn't pinpoint what that energy was, and yet, I knew something was missing.

After my first pole dancing class I knew... and I was hooked... and this too changed my life forever!

As I sat in my first class I proclaimed that I was there to "re-connect with my inner goddess". The ladies had no clue what I was referring to and, at this point, I was very aware of how different I was in this world.

As we sat in a dimly lit studio, no mirrors or candles, we were invited into the slow sensual movements that are the signature S-Factor warm-up.

It was during this first class that I could perceive what I

had been missing for so long. The energy of my female body. The softness, sensuality, strength and fluidity that I had shut down for so long.

I had forsaken my body for my mind and, in that choice, locked up the energy of aliveness and pleasure that my body desired to gift me.

That orgasmic, alive energy was what I allowed myself to have when I danced as a child and in college. I just didn't quite acknowledge that in the past.

As I watched my teacher do a dance to a raunchy, sexy version of one of my favorite songs, my body was suddenly turned on. That joyful, orgasmic, aliveness I had been missing for so long was present and, for the first time in years, I did not judge it.

I allowed myself to be it and I demanded: "I'll have that now please!"

In that moment I became aware that one of the most suppressed energies in my family was that of sexual energy.

We were simply not allowed to have that with our bodies. Our culture, as well as a history of abuse in our family, made this energy forbidden and scary.

This delicious, generative, innate energy is available to all of our bodies from the moment of conception.

I *know* I had it when I was little. I was the exuberance of life. The beauty of childhood expression. Somewhere along the way I let it go in favor of control, conclusions, thoughts, feelings and emotions.

In my very Latin home, we were not allowed to talk about sex, have sex or be sexual. That part of me was squashed very early on. I happened to have created a very beautiful body in this lifetime and most people do not know how to be around me. My father certainly did not know how to deal with all the energy of me and my body.

LETTING GO AND BEING PRESENT WITH THE POLE

The journey with my body and pole dancing is one I speak of often in my work.

In my first book, *Your Body as the Creation of Consciousness*, I wrote:

Over the years, I have learned to listen to my body and be present with her in a whole new way.

Pole dancing gifted me with the chance to let go of my mind and surrender to her.

Surrendering to the way she wants to move, the music she wants to dance to, the moves she wants to make. No matter what they look like!

This didn't happen overnight though. There were many times when I noticed my mind did not want to trust or honor the intelligence of my body.

My mind would say:

"You want me to do what with just one hand?"
"I'm not strong enough to hold myself upside down!"
"Ok, that is crazy, I can't do that!"
"You should not be touching yourself like that."

Musings and lies created by the mind...

There were certain tricks that absolutely required knowing my body would support me and take care of me.

There were so many times when I let go and she surprised

me with total delight.

There were other times when I listened to her and chose to do the trick some other time.

Pole dancing was about tuning in to my body and allowing her to choose what she required in that moment. It was about honoring where she was that day and choosing for her, not against her.

And then, there were the women in my class... the beautiful, courageous women who were on this journey with me. We clapped, cheered and supported each other. We celebrated everything. Nothing was a failure.

How can anything be a failure when you're honoring you?

I was fortunate to have an amazing pole dance teacher. She wasn't just about the fitness part of pole dancing. She had innate healing abilities and spoke to the energies in the room and the energies our bodies were being at the moment.

AND ALONG CAME ACCESS CONSCIOUSNESS®

In 2012, after years of certifications in energy healing, Tantra, QiGong, crystals, oils, nutrition and countless other healing tools, I found the tools of Access Consciousness.

At first, I thought this would be another set of tools I would add to my very large collection. Little did I know this choice would also change my life in a magical way.

It was the difference that Access Consciousness is with the body that created so much more change for me and my body. The tools invite the body to be. We *include* the body in our journey with consciousness. And not in a "you have to eat the right thing" and "work out three times a week" kind of way.

In Access Consciousness, we ask the body questions about anything related to the body. We honor the body's innate wisdom in every choice we make with our bodies.

We are introduced to the idea that the body can and will contribute to your life and living.

Through the Access Consciousness Body Processes, we are able to unlock and unwind the judgments, points of view, decisions and conclusions we have made about our bodies and we invite the magic of our bodies to shine.

Before using these magical tools, I was so shut down with the abuse that I had created in my life that it was challenging for me to even allow anyone to touch me.

Anyone coming into my personal space was a threat. I would shrink and disappear and my barriers would go up immediately.

I remember being at an Access Consciousness 7-Day event in India. My friend Shannon came and sat beside me. I could perceive myself shrinking away. The sensation of contraction was so palpable in my body I was surprised I had never been aware of it before.

As she gently placed her hand on my arm, I said to myself: "Lower your barriers, lower your barriers, breathe, everything is ok. You're safe. Lower your barriers." That was one of the first times I had received kind, gentle touch from a woman.

With these tools, I gained a new sense of awareness with my body. My body was talking to me and I was listening on a whole new level.

I was able to let go of everything I had been holding in my body. Not only for me, but for those my sweet body was trying to heal!

That was another revelation of the contribution our bodies can be... who knew you could have a healing body?! I didn't!!!

When you have a healing body, your body has the capacity to heal others just by being! WHAT?!

I ended up locking things into my body that did not even belong to me because I didn't have this information.

All the abuse the women in my family experienced, the unexpressed rage my father exploded with, the fear my mother lived with, the anxiety my sister experienced.

All of it was *in my body!*

For every sensation I could perceive with my body, I would ask: "Is this mine?" and with the energetic shift of awareness the sensation would dissipate. I would return it to sender with consciousness attached and my body would relax. I would be more open to receiving and more receptive to the information my body was trying to communicate with me.

AND WHAT ABOUT MY DANCING?

HOLY GAMOLIES!!! My dancing changed once I began including the tools of Access Consciousness.

After attending my first Certified Facilitators Training in Venice, Italy, I went to my pole dancing class. After my solo dance, my teacher was amazed at the way my body moved. I was amazed.

That softness, fluidity and femininity I had longed for was finally opening. My body was alive and filled with orgasmic energy. I trusted my body more. I was present with my body in a way I had never been before and it was delicious!

I now had even more awareness with my body. I began to learn so much more about the ways I was being in the world with my body.

The dances showed me the times when I was totally in my head and not present with my body. I saw the ways in which I would give up me in favor of someone else. I learned to listen to my body and the information she was gifting me.

Sex was different too. All that orgasmic energy flowed through me during sex and changed my life and the lives of the men I chose to be with.

Opening to the pleasures of the body had its perks!

THE CONTRIBUTION MY BODY HAS BEEN TO MY LIFE AND LIVING

It was after Venice that I created Pole Dancing For Consciousness™. An Access Consciousness Specialty class designed to invite anyone who chooses it to a different way of moving in the world *with* their bodies.

I went from shy and introverted, to running a global business with clients from all over the world. My body invited me into creating a bigger life with more joy, pleasure and awareness.

If you would have told me five years ago that I would be facilitating men and women into more pleasure and joy with their bodies I would have told you that you were insane!

As a matter of fact, when Pole Dancing For Consciousness™ was born, I thought I was insane! I could not believe that this was flowing through me as one of the ways in which I would contribute to consciousness in the world.

Every day, my body contributes to the creation of my life. As I write this, I've been asking my body what she desires to contribute and the words are flowing out of me as if by magic.

I use the cues my body is giving me to create. The sensations that arise in my body guide me as we create our lives together. Not against each other.

I create my life *with* my body and she is so much happier for it! I am happier for it! Even during those times when I perceive discomfort, I know it's my body trying to communicate something to me.

Move it or lose it!

Back to what I was speaking about in the beginning of this chapter.

I've been traveling for a couple of years focusing on my business. Since my body does not really enjoy "exercising" it was challenging to find places where I could dance.

I've missed dancing and the gift it is to my body.

I've noticed that my strength and flexibility has changed. I've noticed that my body has changed. She's been demanding more movement and more of me.

Gary Douglas, Founder of Access Consciousness, often says: "use it or lose it."

Our bodies are meant for movement, joy, fun and pleasure.

When we don't use them for what they are designed for we lose our communion and connection with them.

I guess my point is, no matter where you are with your body, it's never too late to start. Whether dance or movement are a part of your past or not, there is always today.

Whether you are a professional dancer or not, you *can* find the joy of embodiment through dance.

What may be challenging today will be easy tomorrow!

Our bodies are magic.

And it is my point of view that when we are able to get out of judgment with our bodies and include them in our lives, miracles are available.

Are you willing to discover the magic of your body?

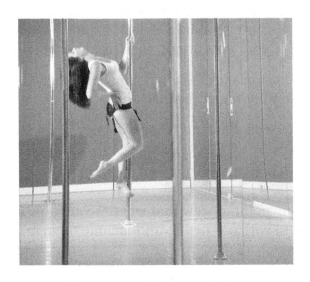

Photo by My Södergren

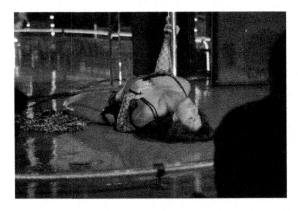

Photo by Kristina Lloyd

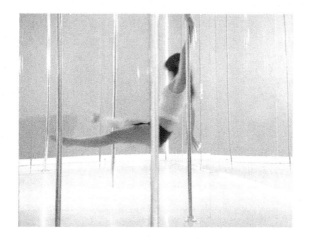

Photo by My Södergren

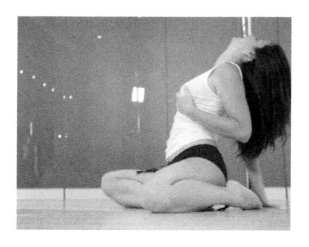

Photo by My Södergren

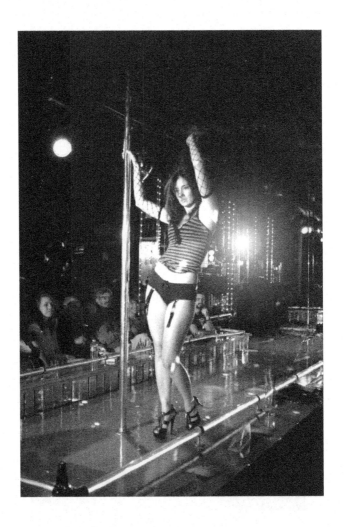

Photo by Kristina Lloyd

Patty Alfonso

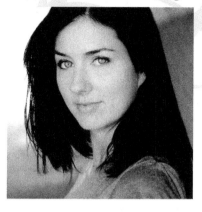

A catalyst for transformation, Patty Alfonso is an internationally acclaimed speaker and an Access Consciousness® Certified Facilitator. She is the author of the #1 International Best Selling Book "Your Body as the Creation of Consciousness™" and the host of the weekly online show *Consciousness is Sexy*.

Patty is a world traveler with a global business that inspires her clients to create magic in their life with their business, their bodies and in their relationships.

She is the creator of Pole Dancing for Consciousness™ and The Essence of You™. Her kind, witty and sharp facilitation invites her clients into having more ease, joy, pleasure and communion.

Born and raised in Guaynabo, Puerto Rico, Patty received her Bachelor's Degree in Sociology from Emory University. She is also certified as a Body/Mind Counselor and Energy Healing Therapist.

For more information about Patty's creations check out:

www.PattyAlfonso.Sexy
www.Consciosuness.Sexy
www.YourBodyIsConsciousness.com
www.PoleDancingForConsciosuness.com

Chapter 2

First, I Danced in Water
By Dr. Glenna Rice

Dancing in water could allude to the primordial sea, to dancing in our mother's womb. It could suggest the waters that birthed us, but that is not what I am referring to.
I danced in the water for many years before I danced on land.

In water is where I began my first intense and magical dance "training" where my body gifted me its love of moving to music, to dancing, to playing with sound and rhythm and choreography.

From the ages of 8-16 I was a synchronized swimmer. I practiced 6 days a week, dancing in the water, no barre, point shoes, or leotard. We were wet, with a suit and a nose clip...and often very oxygen deprived. I loved it!

At 16 it changed. It was no longer fun. Our team was nationally competitive, our coach would become the US Olympic coach, and the first two synchronized swimming Olympic gold medalists swam with me. It had become serious, so much about the competition and control, about being the best and I so hated 6am practice. It didn't work for me anymore ...and maybe, just maybe I had new things to choose and create in my future?

The choice to quit troubled me for many years, but now I can see how this was creating my future from awareness, even if I didn't know that cognitively.

I was willing to let it all go and not hold onto the idea that I should have to continue because I had done it for so long. It was not my thing any longer and letting go allowed something else I enjoyed to show up!

If you are willing to let go of everything then you will allow for greater possibilities and everything around you to contribute to creating your future.

ASK: What are you unwilling to lose that if you did lose it would create a totally new possibility for your future?

Not long after I was hired as an aerobic instructor at a health club. My first job and what crazy fun it was, creating routines, moving to music, sweating and getting paid!

So I am rocking the mid 80's aerobics scene, legwarmers, headbands, Madonna, and Pre Med at the University of Washington and I talk to this girl who tells me about a dance class she is taking for credits.

I am stopped in my tracks! What did she just say? Ballet on campus? A for real class? What? "I WANT THAT!!!!" My whole being screamed!

My dance training on land had begun....

Four days a week I learned ballet and received some great modern and contemporary training. I had walked into a magical wonderland of dance.

The next 6 years, while I completed a degree in Zoology, I took every class I could. Dancing 2-4 hours a day...with rehearsals on the weekends and loved everything about it! My body was so grateful to have this as a contribution to my life.

The things we love to do, that bring us joy, that are easy for us, we can do for hours and never get paid....

We often never acknowledge them for the gift they are and often discount them because they are easy for us. Hard work is what is valued in this reality, not what comes easy.

Your capacities that are easy and joyful, these are the most valuable to this reality, the things that will create money for you if you ask for it. What if you never had to work hard at what you enjoy?

ASK: What have you never acknowledged is easy for you that you pretend you must work hard at so no one, including you, devalues it because it is easy?

"You are unique, and if that is not fulfilled, then something has been lost."
 ~ Martha Graham

MONEY AND DANCE

I was one class short of a degree in dance when I graduated. I was starting graduate school in the fall and I figured, what would I ever do with a degree in dance? You can't make money with dance. This one decision limited what was possible for years.

When I completed graduate school in Physical Therapy I hoped to work with dancers and finding these patients proved to be difficult. Because of this one point of view, you can't make money with dance, I was not able to receive dancers in my practice. They could not even find me. Once you make a decision, nothing that does not match your decisions can you ever be aware of.

When I changed this point of view years later with the tools of Access, not only did I start to have more dancers as well as gymnasts and martial artists in my practice, I also was asked to teach jazz and hip hop classes as a sub when the teachers were out of town. I began to receive money from Dance! Changing this one point of view created a miracle.

ASK: "What decisions about dancing and money have you made that limit the money you can create with dance?"

ACOUSTICAL VIBRATIONS

What is dance? It could be a body's movement with rhythm in space but, that description is missing something.

Does it require music or rhythm? No, as I often find myself dancing in my kitchen with no music on. It is more than bodies moving in space with rhythm. The bodies movement can be created from the music but there is more. What creates dance that is such an invitation to bodies? From classical ballet, dancing with friends at a club, in a class, traditional folk dance or flash mob. When dance pulls you in and makes your body sing, if you are doing it or watching, there is an energy that is created.

> *"We have the capacity to receive messages from the stars and the songs of the night winds."*
> *~ Ruth St. Denis*

The energy of an acoustical vibration. Bodies move with and as the acoustical vibration, and that is what creates the joy of movement that dance is for me.

Dance is the movement of the body that exists in space with an energy that moves the body, inspires the body to move and is created by the body.

An energy of creation and an energy of chaos that allows a joy of movement that is a joy of embodiment. If you allow the body to move with, for and as the acoustical vibration whether the movement is organized into very detailed choreography or ambiguous and undefined then something greater is possible.

This is something we have all perceived and it is never cognitive. The possibility is only limited by our definitions, expectations, projections and judgments about what the dance should be.

When the magic of the movement is there and bodies be that, it creates joy-the joy of having a body and being alive and of living! Bodies love to dance...maybe not all, but if you are reading this, your body probably does.

ASK: How many orders of dance and dancing do I have that keep me and my body from receiving and being the chaos of the acoustical vibration of dance?

PROPRIOCEPTIVE AWARENESS

Proprioceptive awareness is a body's ability to be aware of its relationship in space to everything around it. This is not visual awareness, it is how your body knows its position in space and the position of everything and everyone else, even when you are not looking at them.

It includes more than the 5 senses. Proprioception is the awareness of where your body is in respect to the world around you. This is how your body can learn choreography, follow a teacher, dance with other dancers, balance, turn and leap.

A potent proprioceptive awareness is something that is required for dancers and athletes.

The amazing thing when you are watching dance is the abilities our bodies have to be energetically aware of other bodies dancing, where your body will perceive this magical acoustical vibration in simultaneity.

It is the proprioceptive awareness your body has that allows you to perceive another body moving in space. I can watch dancing on my computer for hours and my body is energized.

When you embody in this reality you embody this entire reality and your body can gift you information about other bodies, the planet and even the universe if you allow it.

An easy practical way to expand your proprioceptive awareness is to increase the awareness of the space between the molecules of your body. Then while keeping that awareness also expand your awareness out to the corners of the room and beyond going out hundreds of miles in all directions or further.

"There are no fixed points in space." ~ Merce Cunningham

This tool to expand your proprioceptive awareness is something you can use to increase your body's ability to balance.

You will find that your body can float on one foot, in pointe shoes, in yoga poses and with turns greater than you could have imagined. It is magic.

The dancers I have shared this with who have used it have told me it is much easier and more effective than the visualization tools they learned in other classes. This tool is dynamic, allowing for more movement while you are balancing. You can be off balance and balance when using this!

Dance is for your body!
How would it like to move?

Without a body, you can't dance. What does it know? Have you ever asked your body?

ASK: Body what do you know that I have been unwilling to listen to?

Dancing for me now is always pleasure and a joy of embodiment for my body, when it is not, I don't do it. This was not always true.

Before I had access to the questions and tools of Access, before I knew I could talk to my body, ask it questions and hear what it knew and was asking for, before I realized that my body is a contribution to my life, living and reality –I would stress out in dance classes.

When I did not get a specific step in class, if I was not "performing" the way I thought I should, I could be very tough on myself and my body and go into such judgement. I would also force my body to class, not knowing that there was a different possibility.

How often have you judged your body for not dancing the way you thought or expected it should? How often have you forced your body to go to class because you should go?

It is so incredibly different now. I have a myriad of questions I can ask while I am dancing and before I go to a class.

If my body is having difficulty with the choreography, I ask my body to contribute. When I ask these questions, every time something magical changes. I move faster, jump higher, turn better. I dance better now than when I was in my 20's and attending class regularly. My body knows what it can do and if I am not stopping it, it always dances better than I can imagine.

ASK: "Body how do you want to do this, how do you want to move?

Then I get out of my body's way and give it permission to move the way it would like to.

ASK "Body duplicate the energy of someone in class that is moving the way you would like to"

It is important that you only ask your body to duplicate the energy of the movement, not the energy of the person.

The person is not something that you want to duplicate, just the energy of their movement. You will be very surprised at how well your body can move when you get out of its way.

Ask Your Body!

To go or not to go? To move or not to move? That is the question. It is always a question for my body not for me.

Like most bodies, my body loves to move and it enjoys different activities on different days. It can choose an intermediate ballet class close to my home that is often challenging, a 5Rythms dance class in a gym where a huge group of people can dance without choreography to amazing music, running to fun music outdoors and swimming.

How do I choose when and what I do? I ask my body.

I travel all over the world and am away from home almost 2 weeks every month, so getting to classes can be a challenge.

When I am home, and there is a class available, I wake up I ask body do you want to go to class today? I always ask my body and I always listen to it.

If it is light, a "yes" I go. If it is heavy or a "no" I don't go, no matter what my point of view is. I have woken up and been so excited for a class because I have not been in a while and my body has surprised me by saying "no".

When it says, "no" I do not go. Every time I was confused by my body's answer something showed up that I was required for, maybe a call I needed to be there for, something with my kids, a different creation.

My body always knew. I trust its awareness and listen to it in everything I do that is for my body, not just dance but what it would like to eat, to wear, who it wants to play with and when and how much it would like to sleep.

When my body says "yes" even if I am tired or incredibly busy, I go to class.

Recently, I was home for a day from traveling in Europe, teaching and attending Access workshops for 15 days straight and had slept very little.

My body bolted out of bed and I heard "I am going to ballet class this morning" and class started in 45 min! I was not interested; it was a new teacher.

I asked my body again, standing up, truth body do you want to go to class this morning and it intensely leaned forward. Of course, I went, my body knew...it was a beautiful class, my body danced superbly and the teacher was a delight.

One way you can ask your body yes and no questions is to stand up and let it know yes is leaning forward and no is leaning backward.

ASK when standing up: Body do you want to do this, eat this, wear this, go to class?

When you include your body and do not force your points of views on it what is created is magic. Creations that are greater than you could imagine!

IT DOESN'T BELONG TO YOU!

When you're having difficulty following the teacher or you are out dancing with your friends and feel foolish ask "Who does this belong to?®"

If anything changes the thought is not yours. Your point of view creates your reality and if you have bought someone else's point of view you will create your reality from their point of view, thinking it is yours.

Nearly all your thoughts, feelings and emotions do not belong to you, you are more psychic than you have ever imagined and are aware of what is going on in other people's heads.

In dance classes, there are a lot of negative thoughts in people's heads. If you can let them go you can begin to dance with more ease and have more space for you.

ASK: How many projections and expectations have you put on your body from other people's points of view that are creating the judgement, separation and rejection of your body from you and you from your body?

How many other people in class are thinking they can't follow the teacher? How many people out dancing at night think they look foolish dancing or have told themselves they can't dance.

It is not yours!

Not long after I learned this tool in an Access class when being a question with everything was still very new to me, I was in a dance performance with quite a large audience.

Back stage, before we were going on, I started to feel incredibly nervous and jittery. My heart was racing and I was no longer present in my body. I started to get a little freaked cause we were about to go on stage, then I remembered the question I had heard in class!

ASK: "Who does this belong to?®"

Instantly, all the "stage fright" was gone and "poof" I was more space than I had ever been before a performance. I went on stage with such ease, truly magical. The ease of the change completely sold me on the question that day and I still use it more than 11 years later.

Before I had this tool, I was so aware of other dancer's thoughts during class and it would often be so loud in my head I would stop what my body could do.

This one tool has given me more freedom in class and allowed a joy with dance I never knew was possible with my body.

Once you are free of all the other people's stuff you are buying as yours you can begin to become aware of what you know and who YOU be. You can begin to ask your body how it would like to move!

If you were to create a reality that worked for you, what would it include, what would you create?

Enjoy the Dance!

Dr. Glenna Rice

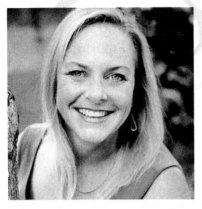

Dr. Glenna Rice, DPT is a Physical Therapist, a Access Consciousness® Certified Facilitator, Access Body Class Facilitator, co-creator of The Energetic Synthesis of Structural Embodiment, owner of Access Physical Therapy in San Rafael, CA and a contributing author in two bestselling books on parenting.

Glenna travels internationally, facilitating workshops to create greater awareness with bodies and anything participants are asking to change.

Glenna is also a single mother of three, who was able to negotiate raising incredible children on her own without having to be a perfect mom. Glenna teaches Conscious Parenting Conscious Kids classes worldwide and has a monthly radio show The Questionable Parent.

For more information go to:

www.glennarice.com

www.drglennarice.accessconsciousness.com

You can find her on Facebook as Dr. Glenna Rice, DPT, and listen to her on Soundcloud at soundcloud.com/glenna-rice and The Questionable Parent at thedrpatshow.com.

Chapter 3

Magical Moving Molecules:
From Cripple to Dancer
By Merlijn Wolsink

DANCE... what is there not to say about it? There is so much and way more than I can put down here, yet I'd love to invite you to a little of what I've come to know and experience.

I love movement. I love bodies.

Moving my body and dancing brings me 'down to earth'. It inspires me to be here, it gets me out of my head, into my body and into embodiment, which includes everything on this planet.

Dancing and movement allow me to be the space that allows miracles to occur.

My reality with dance, movement and my body has had many colors throughout my entire life. It did not start from a desire to dance and I've not always been best friends with my body.

I used to perform, play, and go crazy in front of my family. I'd put some music on and arrange my family in the living room so they could watch my performance.

The safe space of my family allowed that, and I wasn't made wrong for it. The occasional visitor that would come along: "That's weird, he's wearing a wig and a dress and is dancing to music and singing like Snow White and the

Little Mermaid."

Yes, that was me. I loved moving like a princess with weird arm gestures combined with musical tunes and melodies.

FANTASY INTO REALITY

I used music and fairy tales to escape reality, because I enjoyed that so much more. It gave me a different sense of life here.

I was a dreamer and I lived in my own magical world of Disney movies, creative outbursts and dance. In the outside world I felt like such a weirdo most of the time and now I know, I was extremely aware of everything and everyone around me.

As a kid I walked on my toes and I was more outside of my body than really embodied. My mom noticed that every time I would dance to music I was much more coordinated than in gym class at school.

She asked if I wanted to join ballet class, as she knew that it might be a good idea for me to get a greater sense and connection with my body. It could get me a little more 'down to earth', instead of always floating around in different spaces and not being present here and now.

So I took ballet, and it was fun playing with all the girls in class. My ballet teacher said, "We'll make you very flexible!" That excited me and I thought "Oh! Is that possible?"

FOR THE LOVE OF MUSICALS!

My parents took me to see CATS the musical. I was enchanted by all the things I saw and not necessarily by the dancers dancing. It was more the combination of all the elements coming together as a full theatre production.

The apparent richness, the movement and dynamic energy of everything that comes along with theatre was something that intrigued me. Costumes, lights, the set, the actors, dancers, makeup, wigs, music and loud drums, going through the whole room and making me and my body... MOVE. I felt it in my entire body.

Music and singing was what appealed to me most. Snow White's high notes came effortlessly out of my boy soprano throat and I loved listening to the harmonies of our family choir, conducted by my grandfather.

It was always difficult to listen to them and sit down and sit still. Mostly I would move around the room doing other things while still being extremely connected and aware of the music and the harmonies. With very sharp ears, I had pitch-perfect hearing. Music inspired me to move, and always got me moving.

Whether it was my vocal chords or the rest of my body, it always allowed me to connect to greater energies, more lightness, inspiration, more being.

PUTTING ON THE DANCING SHOES

After being in 'regular' schools, feeling like a weirdo and being bullied for long enough, I wanted more creativity in my life.

I chose to go study vocals and piano as a music student at the high school for music and dance. That felt like more fun.

After being there for a year and seeing more dance and musical theatre, I realized that if I wanted to perform in musicals I had to work on my body. I also needed to work on my dance technique and skills to be able to join the chorus line of the ensemble. I wanted to do everything on that stage. And so I did.

An intense journey of training myself to become a dancer started. After a year of dance pre-education and some extra classes each week, I was accepted to the Rotterdam Dance Academy (Codarts) in the Netherlands, a school that is known for delivering dancers with a high level of contemporary and classical technique.

SHAPESHIFTING – CREATING MY BODY

"What was in your mind, your hands created; that was your reality," is how my mom describes me as a kid.

That was true. Whether it was a clay doll, a miniature set for all my Disney play figures, a costume or some other 3D creation...when I had something in mind that I truly wanted, I made it. There was no doubt in my world. I could do it.

The same applied when I started dancing. During my first classes and auditions I was told, "We are not sure if you will make it through dance school, let alone have a professional career in dance."

They said, "Your charisma is fantastic but your body is simply not good enough; you are not turned out and you are not flexible enough." I was like: "Well, can I train in that? Can I stretch my muscles? Improve my technique? That's what school is for, right?" I went for it and did everything in my power to prove that I could do it.

My body changed, my posture changed and my muscles and joints became more flexible and strong. Soon I had all sorts of internships with several dance companies and I kept on WOWing the school board during all of that. I even went to New York on a Fullbright Scholarship.

One of my capacities as a shapeshifter is that I can look at the dancers and people who inspire me, people who have something that I want to have and be as well, and after a while my body starts to be like that too.

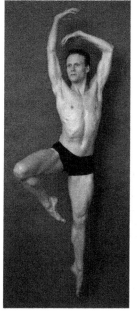

Looking back at my career, I have always been able to create my body shape and train it into everything that was required for all the many different dances and theatre jobs I had.

For all the technical contemporary work, I developed big muscled and flexible legs.

With CATS I eventually moved like a cat. With LA CAGE AUX FOLLES I could fall into a split every single show, or move like a monkey in WICKED or like a cool Jet in WEST SIDE STORY...

And my voice would also shift along through all the ranges that the various roles demanded of me.

My body always changed fast, responding to the energy that I tapped into. Sometimes it was tough. On top of all the creation and inspiration were all the judgments that my body wasn't good enough, that I would never be good enough or that something was wrong.

I was often frustrated,
with myself and with my body.

As I desired more and more and when the 'magic' I knew was possible didn't show up fast enough... I would curse my body.

Have you ever done that? Judge your body to the point where all your space was just FULL of judgment?

That created a lot of stress in my body. Lots of feelings got jammed up, creating a big build-up of energy that often created the moment where I would explode, get stuck and want to stop everything...

If only I knew a little more then of what I know now! The fact that judgments... are not actually real. They are made up.

What if judgment with your body is something you can choose, or not? We are taught to judge.

I had a lot of unconsciousness around this. I simply could not manage all the thoughts, feelings and emotions that were going on, while changing physically and psychologically and having HUGE awarenesses of everything around me. My sweet body acted it all out.

Somewhere, below all the frustration, there was always that strong spark and knowing that this was just a moment we were going through. That something greater was available and that more magic was possible...

STEPPING INTO THE WORLD OF ACCESS CONSCIOUSNESS®

I came across Access Consciousness when I was doing the musical theatre show called WICKED, a show about magic. How funny the way consciousness works!

First, I didn't want to know about Access Consciousness. The Clearing Statement® - a tool we use to change the energies and clear judgment - sounded way too weird to me.

My head and body were so full of fight, stress, anxiety,

frustration and everything that wasn't mine, there was simply no space for me to allow the tools into my world.

I was working hard enough to perform at my best every night while still feeling so unhappy.

When the same feelings and emotions kept on coming up again and again, my mom asked if I wished to let it all go... and I said "YES!" and she ran the Access Consciousness Clearing Statement.

I was somewhat dazzled and asked "Is that that thing that I didn't want you to use on me?!" She said, "Yes, I'm sorry!"

I went shopping and realized that within 10 minutes all the misery was gone. It had cleared and disappeared. "Wow... what the f***?!"

I had been carrying that energy for months and years, trying to change it, shift it, figure it out and solve it. Now I felt light and my body felt light. I had space again to breathe. I could relax.

So much information and possibilities followed when I started listening to some Access Consciousness seminars by Dr. Dain Heer and then, I took the core classes.

Every class I took allowed me to be greater and keep growing and expanding. I kept letting go of layers of shit. I kept unraveling the true Being: ME.

The tools allowed me to start creating more freedom and possibility and to be even greater, whatever that was...

I started to see what's actually great about me and my body and how much of the insanity of this reality was never mine. I knew again that I could create with all the cells and molecules in my body.

DEALING WITH PAIN AND INJURIES

I've had lots of injuries along the way. Most likely due to forcing my body to do certain things that it wasn't ready for at the time. Before Access Consciousness, I didn't have the tools to create *with* my body.

It starts with a muscle twitch, snap, tear, break or an awareness that 'sneaks' in, which develops into 'pain'.

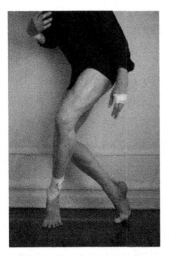

Then you start trying to figure out what is 'wrong'. You try to fix it, and with every attempt, with every person you visit, more projections are added, adding to the charged energy, contraction and stuckness.

Most of the discomforts were actually my body changing to keep up with the way I was changing... a talent our bodies are SO capable of doing.

Only when you add a judgment to that change do you solidify it into an injury. The judgment defines a changing and transforming muscle as 'muscle pain' instead of a 'changing muscle'.

Funny how we use words to create 'pain' instead of receiving the awareness of something changing in our bodies.

Every physical challenge inspired me to learn more about anatomy, icing, stretching and strengthening. I tried different tools and techniques to increase my body's recovery speed.

I've learned so much more from listening to my body and receiving its information while using the tools of Access

Consciousness. They inspire a unique way of being with your body and I was curious and excited about what I could change with my body.

If only I had known I didn't have to create all those injuries and complaints!

CREATING WITH THE MOVING, MAGICAL MOLECULES OF MY BODY

The tools of Access Consciousness added a whole different depth and breadth to my experience of injury. They changed the way I am with my body. They expanded the possibilities of everything I already knew and used!

What if beneath every 'weakness', pain and injury, beneath every judgment you have about yourself and your body, there is actually a great knowing, awareness and magical power?

What if all the molecules in your body are actually moving all the time? What if nothing in your body is ever *not* moving? Even as you asleep?

It's like... MAGIC. It changes a LOT for people when they realize this, especially when they think their body is 'stuck' or 'broken'.

Before Access Consciousness, lots of physical therapists and body workers could help me heal an injury but, eventually, it would come back. As if the cells would immediately recreate the trauma again when triggered.

IT ALL STARTED CHANGING

What if the molecules and cells of our bodies actually respond to the energy they are surrounded by?

Our cells and molecules respond to our thoughts,

feelings, emotions and surroundings. What if you could communicate with all of them?

How much space can you be and give every molecule to move freely?

With the energetic tools of Access Consciousness, I instantly noticed a huge shift and change in my movement.

As soon as I started dropping the judgment, expanding the space between the molecules of my body, lowering my energetic barriers, destroying and uncreating points of view, returning energies to sender things literally started moving.

My legs would fly with ease, I could add weights to my work out, stretching became more dynamic, and moving through the space became safe and free.

Acknowledging my body and its consciousness and asking it questions made things a whole lot more fun:

Hey body, let's play... how about... four turns?

How much ease and joy can we have performing this choreography?

Which exercise first?

How can this work out better than we ever imagined possible?

When you ask questions, you begin creating *with* your body to become even greater whatever way IS possible!

Most of us ambitious dancers and movers know that deep down inside, we start forcing the change. Pushing ourselves through self-judgment by what we are told or taught to do by our teachers, mentors and choreographers.

My body required a major unlocking from judgment, for it to be free and move naturally.

What absolutely rocked my world were the Access Consciousness Body Processes® I received in my first Foundation Class. I ran them on myself and changed my hamstring injuries, bruises and old scar tissue.

I remember the moments, full of amazement, when I would run a simple energetic process and rapidly feel the muscles, tissues and even tendons change, move and heal.

It was like a mini earthquake was going on under my own hands. Everything moving back to its original place or better. Some injuries were over 10 years old!

I got in touch with my body in a completely different way. I felt whole with my body and I could receive it more and more.

Not only did my reality with my body change: my life lit UP. It had always been true to me that this was possible and I finally had the tools to do it. And BE it.

If only all dancers, athletes, physical therapists and body workers would know about this. Everyone's life and body would be so different!

Pains that couldn't change, according to the "body experts," really weren't what they seemed to be. When adding the body's consciousness and awareness to it was a whole different story!

Of course, I still visit massage therapists or other body workers to care for my body, only now it is a choice, not a necessity or a way to survive.

I'm thriving and it's by choice.

I was always a dynamic performer and the Access

Consciousness tools allowed me to become even greater. I wish that for everyone, for every body.

It's such a gift to not need to control your body. To discover the possibilities of creating with it, with consciousness. Magical..."OMG, I can talk to the cells in my body and they change by my request! WHAT?!"

I was taught: "Technique and control over your body gives you freedom to dance." Energetic creation with your body gives you even *more* freedom than just technique.

What if 'having control over your body' could be more about having an awareness, a connection, a communion with every molecule of your body?

What if that allows you to co-create with him/her?

What if when you move, be, dance, change - embracing all of you and your body exactly as you are – it leads you to being greater?

INSPIRING OTHERS TO DISCOVER THEIR MAGIC

After thoroughly discovering magic with my own body, many other bodies followed. I started to apply these tools in my classes with my students and the people I worked with in one-on-one sessions.

Results were miraculous with the basic Access Consciousness tools, the verbal processing and body processes. I have facilitated many acute bone fractures or broken bones that would not heal and changed all sorts of injuries with many people.

I created a class "Magic with Pain and Injuries" which is a true joy to facilitate. Seeing ordinary people, as well as dancers and physical therapists, experience the amazement with their bodies that I had as well.

When I work with bodies now, I always use questions and have a conversation with the bodies I work with, including my own.

Your body has its own consciousness.

Every molecule in the Universe has consciousness, which is what makes the Universe such an abundant place to live in!

I started using questions in my dance and theatre classes or when I would lead rehearsals. Most dancers had the same skepticism as I had when I first heard about the Access Consciousness tools.

Applying the tools - destroying and uncreating points of view, asking questions and expanding the energy and space between the molecules - all created magic in the classroom.

Bodies and voices responded and the performers noticed it. I receive many, many thank you's for how these fairly simple, yet super effective tools have such a great impact on the creation of their whole life and body. They also get the jobs they really desire!!

When I facilitate a movement class and I include the bodies in creation of the class, change happens faster.

When people gain the trust that their body knows so much about movement, energy, receiving, awareness and creation, it's truly beautiful to see and experience.

It touches me every time how grateful people are to discover their *own magic*, both during classes and afterwards.

As co-host of the *Conscious Body Movement* radio show together with Greg Dyer, a dear friend and personal trainer from the United States, we've been able to explore many different things with movement and bodies. What else is possible for more bliss in embodiment? It is a truly great adventure that has inspired so many people. I am so grateful!

BEING CLOUDED BY JUDGMENT

How come we don't always experience that abundant magic in our lives and with our bodies?

We are taught to judge everything constantly. We function from a lot of conclusions and unconsciousness with our bodies, which stops everything else we could be, do, have or receive dead in it's tracks. What else is possible?®

I went to see a massage therapist once. Lying on her massage table I was complaining about my aches and pains and then she asked me "Do you realize what all these cells have done for you? Could you be grateful for them instead of being so hard on them?"

I was baffled! I had made my body wrong for so long I had gotten used to it!

What if you can be grateful for all the cells and molecules in your body?

Our bodies are magnificent. What would happen if we stopped judging them and have more allowance and gratitude?

Thank you, body!

FROM WEAKNESS TO GREATNESS

Before I started dancing I was called a 'cripple'. I had an extremely weird body posture. A pelvis that was tucked under, my arms were crooked and over-turned out from the shoulders, and the shoulder heads were rotated forward onto my ribcage. Not a standard dancer-body to say the least and 'wrong' in so many ways.

Someone who inspired me hugely is choreographer Bob Fosse. He created his dance style from his own physique and choreographed shows and movies like *Cabaret* and *Sweet Charity*.

His body and hips were turned in, his back was hunched, he had thin hair and he didn't like his hands. His style is more Jazz and Vaudeville and he always used the weird and odd angles of the body while still making it look elegant and sensual.

Basically, he turned his apparent 'weaknesses' into greatness with his signature moves like pigeon-toed feet,

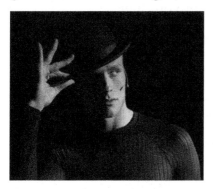

back bumps, waterfall arms, drooping shoulders and spiked teacup fingers.

"I put my body to work in a different way so it is fun to watch" quoting Mr. Fosse.

I could SO relate to it all!

His difference, his 'not normal' and still looking amazing inspired me.

When I saw the dancers perform in a production of Chicago, I was like "YES! THAT! That is what I want to dance and work with". And I did. I was hired to be a part of and to supervise a national tour of *Chicago*.

A DIFFERENT POINT OF VIEW

During most of my early years in dance school my arms were often judged as "crooked", "droopy" and "not right."

59

One of my dance teachers even called me a "gnarly olive tree."

I had totally bought the belief that my arms were ugly. A belief I used to not stretch out, not be different, not stand out. I didn't fit the school's standards.

During a Musical Theater Dance program at Jacob's Pillow, choreographer Chet Walker asked me, "Why don't you fully stretch your arms out?" My response was, "Because they are crooked and they look weird." He said, "Merlijn, you have such amazing, long and beautiful arms, you should use them."

He showed me a different point of view that totally changed my life and the way my body moved, that went beyond judgment into greatness. He opened the door to greatness for me just a little, so grateful for you Chet.

IS THIS ACTUALLY MINE? – TALKING BODIES

Body awareness can result in many different things if not acknowledged as body awareness. I've had lots of 'complaints' in my body that were unexplainable.

One of them was in New York City when I was attending a semester at the Alvin Ailey School. I ended up having an inflammation in my left Achilles tendon.

It just showed up and I had no logical medical reason or reference point as to how exactly it had occurred. After about three weeks, three more students were sitting with me at the side of the classroom, all with an Achilles inflammation in the left leg and no one could figure it out, including the physical therapy office.

Was this actually ours to start with?
Who did that belong to?

Of course I could mention lots of medical, linear and cognitive reasons for how this 'happened' or got created, and it might be different for everyone.

Yet, bodies 'talk' and communicate with each other, they are aware and have the capacity to adapt to their environment, to create and show you what they are aware of.

Would we have even created this Achilles tendinitis if we would have acknowledged that our bodies were aware of one another? That something we feel in our body, is not necessarily ours to start with?

Asking, "Who does this belong to?®" for everything I notice in my body has absolutely changed my life. It just acknowledges how aware my body and I actually are.

MORE OF THAT PLEASE!

How cool is it that our bodies are so aware?

What if it's possible to create with that awareness and use it to your advantage? I actually use my body to receive information about the bodies I am working with, especially in class and in sessions. And I use this awareness to create my own life and body... When I'm aware of a body or an energy that inspires me and what I like more of for myself I ask: "More of that please!" I still do this in the gym or in the classroom.

You don't want to duplicate other bodies and people's points of view, you want to extrapolate the energy, space and consciousness so you and your body can use it to create and re-arrange all the molecules of your life and body.

Everything can be a contribution if you are willing to receive the awareness and choose what works for you and what you would like to add to your life. It can be a lot of fun, and you can always add to it or let go of what doesn't work for you!

Instant creation with my body

Recently I took a dance class and ended up applying the tools that I teach in my Pain and Injury Class and Movement Class on myself.

I kicked a little higher than my muscles could stretch in those 10 seconds and it HURT. I instantaneously applied the tools: I used the Access Consciousness Clearing Statement on my points of view, judgments, conclusions, past experiences and trauma. I expanded my space and the space between the molecules and chose to not buy that it was going to be an injury. It changed. Molecules shifted. I asked:

> What energy can I be here?
>
> Body, what do you require?
>
> What energy, space and consciousness can me and my body be?

I stopped for a moment in class to do this. I felt all of it change, and within 2 minutes I joined class again.

It kept on changing and moving throughout the class and I did some gentle stretching and processing after that.

At night, the trauma was gone, how cool is that?

Joy and body loving

So much of the moments in my dancer and theatre life were so amazing, and I could not always receive the gift and power of it at that time. All of the judgments were in the way, clouding all the joy.

Joy can exist if you stop judging negatively and maybe even positively. You don't even need to 'accept' yourself or your body to be in allowance of all of you and to receive and embrace all of you.

If you go and look through your own life... how much experiences with your body have you had that were actually GREAT?

Truly enjoying your body without a point of view? Have you ever truly acknowledged, embraced and received it?

What if JOY could be your reality with your body?

Your body is still here as you are reading this right now. It's lived and created with you through it all. If you would embrace and receive all the molecules of your body, what else is possible for your life?

What can we all contribute to more pleasure, creation and magic with dance, movement and with our bodies?

What else is possible we haven't considered yet?

GRATITUDE

Facilitating Access Consciousness classes and using the tools with people is such a gift – I get to see everyone's own light turn on!

Every single time I facilitate this work, I become greater and receive so much from it myself.

I'm so grateful to everyone and everything that has contributed to my life and career, that has chosen to work and play with me and has inspired me to be me.

Thank you Patty Alfonso for inviting me to be part of this

amazing creation.

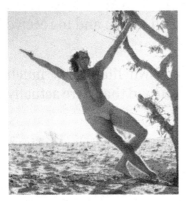

And of course, thank you Gary Douglas and Dr. Dain Heer for creating Access Consciousness and all the life-changing tools.

And thank you to my best friend: my sweet body.

I'm so grateful for you and our ability to move, dance, breathe and live.

Merlijn Wolsink

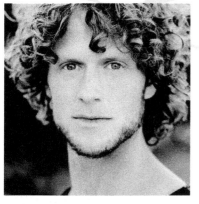

Artist. Dancer. Speaker. Body Magician

Born in The Netherlands, Merlijn Wolsink is internationally known for his kindness, gentleness energetic, potent and life-changing facilitation. His 15 years of professional experience includes: dance, movement, voice, music, stretching, the pragmatics of awareness, well-being of mind, spirit and body.

Merlijn invites people to their own greatness. His light, fun, practical and magical approach has inspired many people to have more allowance and kindness with their bodies.

Merlijn is an Access Consciousness® Certified Facilitator. He facilitates classes, sessions, and workshops, including his Specialty Classes: Magic with Pain and Injuries and The Magic of Moving Your Body.

For more about Merlijn classes you can go to:

www.merlijnwolsink.nl
www.merlijnwolsink.accessconsciousness.com
www.merlijnwolsinkblog.com

You can contact Merlijn on social media or shoot him an email at merlijn@handsonaccess.nl.

Chapter 4

Dancing as My Therapy
By Amy Shine

As far back as I can remember, I have always been fascinated not just by dance, but by all movement. I grew up in Ireland so the only real dance class available to me was Irish Dancing.

I went to classes for a few months and although I was good at it, the training frustrated me. It was so restrictive. With Irish dancing, you cannot move your hands and your upper body doesn't move. So after a few months, I got bored and quit!

When I got to primary school (middle school) there were two forms of movement available to girls: basketball and running. I was actually good at running so I pursued athletics for a few years. As I hit puberty, boys and friends distracted me and it wasn't until my early 20s that I discovered my buried love for dance again.

THE BEGINNING OF FINDING DANCE AS AN ESCAPE

When I was 20, I took off to Ibiza (Balearic Islands of Spain) for a summer, working holiday. Ibiza is home of the greatest clubbing experiences in the world.

It was here on this mystical island, in these world famous nightclubs, that I discovered what a release dance was for me.

Even though I was living on this magical island for a summer, I was still so lost, so confused and carrying around a lot of pain inside me.

A couple of years previous, my oldest brother was killed in a car accident and it had left so much sadness and grief in our family. My close relationship to my other brother, who was still alive, had fallen apart. I found myself with so much anger and sorrow. I honestly did not know what to do with it.

The clubs in Ibiza were alive and vibrant. When I danced, I escaped from reality with the movement and the music. I partied a lot that summer and continued until the next summer.

This world baffled me and I was totally dissatisfied by it. Things I was supposed to care about like finding a partner, getting married, going to college, having a career, were not enough for me. I always had a sense that there HAD to be more.

BREAKING DOWN OR BREAKING THROUGH?

After two summers of partying, dancing in clubs and drinking more than my small body could handle, it all began to fall apart. I fell apart. I had a total nervous breakdown. It was scary for my family to see. To the so-called professionals in this world who like to give labels, I was psychotic!

To me, I was actually seeing a totally different world. I could see things that no one else could see and hear things that no one else could hear.

While this world called it a 'breakdown', I can see now it was a 'breakthrough'. My life as I knew it would never be the same. I would never be the same.

During this breakdown, all I kept hearing was how I had to pursue Yoga, dance, meditation, and bodywork. I was getting all this information about schools, children, healing centers and consciousness.

There were times during this period where I was awake and alive. I knew that I was here for something different. There were also times where my mind was so intense and dark that I just wanted to die.

It was such a struggle at the start. I was put on medication that totally numbed every feeling in my body. I literally felt nothing. I was totally dead inside. I couldn't laugh. I couldn't dance. I had no friends. I literally spent all my time with my family. I was so grateful for them and their kindness.

I couldn't finish my last year in college. I was 21 and going to a counselor who told me I needed to go to a 12-step recovery program. When I woke up every day, I wished that I wasn't in this world anymore. Yet, I knew I was here for another reason and I needed to stay here and get better.

I took a local office job, which I hated. I struggled every day to stay awake at the computer as the medication made me so sleepy. It took all my energy, but I did whatever I could to help me get better. I took Yoga classes and went to Medjugorje with my mother, looking for something there to fix me. I tried pretty much anything while all the time struggling with the demons in my head.

I started to go to 12-step recovery meetings in my local hometown. I was so depressed and didn't know if I would ever enjoy living again.

The people at these meetings were different. They were so kind. They talked about having racing minds, feeling lost, destroyed, like they had nothing. They also talked about how they recovered and changed. Their lives were now joyful again.

These meetings gave me hope, and for the first time I didn't feel so alone. I didn't feel so crazy and I was seeing how I wasn't the only person who was battling demons.

These meetings were a central part of my life for five years and I will be forever grateful for the people I met in those rooms. They were truly some of the kindest and most caring people in the world.

One day I was talking to one of the members. I was mourning the fact that I was a 23-year-old girl who loved to dance and, since I could no longer drink, going out to nightclubs no longer appealed to me. He suggested I try 5 Rhythms Dancing and so I did!

THE BEGINNING OF DANCE
AS A TRANSFORMATIONAL TOOL

I will never forget the first 5 Rhythms class I took. I danced around the room that night with so much joy. This was it. I knew this was possible! I could actually have a space to dance and be free and let go in an environment where there was no drinking or drugs.

This began my journey in using dance as a form of therapy. For two years, I went to every 5 Rhythms class and workshop. It was so much more than dancing. It was therapy. We used our breath. We connected with each other.

We went from flowing around the room, feeling a bit self-conscious and in our heads, to letting ourselves be chaotic and letting go of everything in our minds, being totally free and dancing like no one is watching.

It was everything I was looking for when I was clubbing in Ibiza, except now I was doing it in a safe environment and totally sober. It was alive, vibrating, euphoric, ecstatic, healing and restorative.

Unlike in Ibiza, when I would have the high followed by a massive come down, this movement left me feeling like I had more of me.

These classes opened my whole world. I became so open to connecting and dancing with people from all different walks of life. All the walls of separation we put up between each other, just fell away.

The dance would bring me through so many emotions and energies: frustration, anxiety, racing mind, and anger to ease, gratitude and joy.

Memories from the past would surface during the classes and I would just move with the energies. Just like magic, the memories in my mind would leave.

I truly know that there was so much transformational healing for me in those classes. I also accessed a joy that my previous life and the medication had killed.

The best gift was the knowing that I no longer needed drugs and alcohol to have that joy and ecstasy that I chased so much in Ibiza. Now I had ME and I had dance, and this world could not ever take that from me again.

CREATING MY DREAMS:
FACILITATING A DANCE MOVEMENT GROUP

I was so inspired from the dance and the power of movement in my life that I did my college thesis on: "The value of dance movement as a therapy for women in recovery from addiction."

I invited six women who were part of the 12-step program to be part of a monthly dance movement group. This was a game changer.

"And those who were seen dancing
Were thought to be insane
by those who could not hear the music."
~ Friedrich Nietzsche

We all transformed in this group. I got to facilitate these amazing ladies from uncomfortableness, awkwardness, fear, anger, and frustration into laughter, joy, fun and letting crap go.

We created something very special together. We bonded, we laughed, we danced, we cried, we sang and we changed. To this day, this experience shaped me in so many ways.

I saw the power in movement not just for me but for these women. One participant went from being on numbing medication, feeling alone and isolated, to dropping the dosage of her medication, finding friendship, laughter and dance through the group.

The transformation of all the participants in this group was profound. At the start of every class, everyone reported a mix of different resistances and barriers such as anxiety, self-consciousness, shyness, crankiness and not wanting to move.

Once we started to move our bodies, there was a shift from the mind state to a presence in the body and a release of emotions.

As we moved, danced, stayed aware and present, we also let go of all judgments and thoughts. There was a level of joy that we all accessed in these classes with ourselves, our bodies and everyone else.

In the end, through this movement, we were all able to access parts and pieces of ourselves that we had lost: our imaginations, sense of wonder and curiosity, childlike play, joy, potency, and our connection to our bodies.

This was the art of transforming and healing through Dance.

DANCE AS THE BODY OF CONSCIOUSNESS

It was evident for me from my own personal experience and from this group that something else was happening here.

Through dance we were accessing our consciousness with our bodies. It was undeniable. We were no longer using substances to get that high. Instead, we were experiencing a joy with our bodies. All our walls, barriers and judgments that were creating all the unconsciousness in our body would melt away when we danced. In that space we accessed a sense of oneness, connection to ourselves and something greater within us.

As Gary Douglas, Founder of Access Consciousness® states: "Consciousness is the ability to be present in your life in every moment, without judgment of you or anyone else. It is the ability to receive everything, reject nothing, and create everything you desire in life – greater than what you currently have, and more than what you can imagine."

THE BODY REMEMBERS

Through my research, I have found lots of evidence to support what I already knew and was experiencing through dance.

Our bodies were so much more than just bones and muscle. Our bodies have cells that store all the memories of our past. Through movement and other mediums like the Access Consciousness Body Processes, we can release the past and create new pathways.

> *"The whole history of a person is contained within the physical structure therefore traumatic events cause muscular contractions in the organisms that restrict the flow of energy."*
> *~ Wilhelm Reich*

Neuroscience shows that the right hemisphere of the brain is interacting with the limbic system and a direct map of the state of the body is stored in the brain.

In Pylvanainen's research paper, Shuren and Graftman state that the right hemisphere stores representations of emotions associated with past experiences and when an individual encounters a similar scenario in the present, the emotional experiences of the past are retrieved from the brain.

If difficult emotions are encountered, like anger or anxiety, when the body is activated into movement, the state in the body and the brain change which can then change the mood.

We can actually change our destructive reaction patterns, behaviors and response systems and create healthier pathways in our brains. We then store that in our bodies and that will result in a lasting change!

*"When you have movement of energy,
you have change."
~ Dr. Dain Heer
Co-Creator of Access Consciousness*

MY DISCOVERY OF ACCESS CONSCIOUSNESS

Personally, I had experienced a lot of change in my mindset and body from dancing. I had a lot more joy and hope. Yet, there were still a lot of emotional rollercoasters for me.

I would have days of feeling great and the next day I would be on the floor, overwhelmed with sadness and emotions, not wanting to be in the world.

I just knew there had to be an easier way. There had to be something else. My beautiful friend Rachael O'Brien was doing this thing called Access Consciousness.

I could see from being around her that she had a lot more joy and ease and was not as emotional as she used to be!

I took the Access Bars® class and my whole world opened. It was light bulbs in my head going off everywhere, everything falling into place.

I had spent the previous five years believing I was so wrong, and that I had an incurable disease of the mind.

In that class, everything changed. I woke up and had this massive awareness that it was all LIES!! That there was NOTHING wrong with me!

Judgment kills our bodies. Judgment is always a lie and it kills the creation of your life. I had been in so much judgment of myself. Getting your Bars run literally starts to dissipate the electromagnetic charge on all our thoughts, ideas and emotions. Mainly we let go of our JUDGMENTS.

As a serial self-judger, getting my Bars run and having all these judgments literally deleted from my brain and body, opened a whole new world for me.

Now, that I was getting the judgments out of the way, nothing could stop me and so began the creation of my life.

I took all the classes I could and I quickly took all the tools of Access Consciousness and started to apply them to my life.

*"If you get over your judgments:
The miracle of you will instantly BE."
~ Dr. Dain Heer
Co-Founder of Access Consciousness*

CREATING MY LIFE
WITH ACCESS CONSCIOUSNESS AND DANCE

My first creation with the tools of Access Consciousness and what I knew about dance was the basis of the creation of 'Shine Movements'.

It's an invitation for people to have fun with their bodies, dance and experience joy again. If you tell me you can't dance, or have no rhythm, then I'd like to work with you!

Dancing isn't about looking a certain way or following the steps. Dancing is a form of movement. If you are moving, you are dancing.

When you let your body move in whatever way it desires, with no form, no structure, and beyond the judgments in your head about what it looks like, something magical happens.

Everything in your head is lies and designed to limit you. This reality is designed to keep you in a box and controlled.

Dance is a judgeable offense here in this reality. When you are willing to dance with no judgment and with no form or structure, you become uncontrollable by this reality! You step out of the box!

I like to move people beyond the lies so they can access the joy of embodiment and this in turn can transform your body, relationships, and your life.

Movement and dance combined with the Access Consciousness questions and clearing statements are profound when used together.

WAKE UP AND MOVE

When I wake in the morning, there's sometimes a density in my head and my body. In Access Consciousness, we talk about how 99 percent of your thoughts, feelings and emotions are not yours!

You can ask: What am I aware of? Is this mine? Or someone else's? And return to sender anything that doesn't belong to you, with consciousness attached.

Get moving! I dance everywhere. In my garden, on the beach, by the pool outside my house. If I was feeling heavy or sad, I would put my headphones on, go find a space to dance, and let my body move and be free.

Within minutes, the heaviness and sadness would lift and I would be energized, joyful and have a sense of me again.

That is the power of movement, my friends.

Dance first. Think Later.

You don't have to get to a class. You can put some music on

in your house and dance there. You can also do 10 minutes of stretching.

All it takes is a few minutes of moving to totally shift your energy from tired, heavy, and cranky to awake, alive and energized.

Get moving, get dancing and see what happens!

*"If you are always trying
to be normal, you will never know
how amazing you can be."
~ Maya Angelou*

Dancing with Kids

I've been working with kids and young people for a few years now, bringing movement, yoga and energy work to their lives.

I'm not interested too much in teaching them dance routines. Routines just get them to mimic my movements and give them a reason to judge themselves for not doing it right.

I desire more. I desire to create a change in their worlds and to empower them.

I ask lots of questions:

What can we create together?

What do these kids desire?

What would be fun for them?

What can I contribute to them and what could they contribute to me?

Every day before I go to a class, I ask:

What energy space and consciousness can me and my body be, to be the energy, space and consciousness that they require?

Every day before I go to a class, I destroy and un-create all my decisions, judgments and conclusions about me, about the class, about the students and any conclusions I have about what the class has to look like.

This creates the space for the magic of possibilities to show up. Rather than telling them what to do or forcing them to follow me, I ask them to create dances and their own movement with me.

I invite them to be the teacher. I invite them to have fun and joy with movement. I invite them not to judge or compare themselves to anyone. When given the freedom to express themselves and create: these kids and young people create magic.

THE TOOLS OF ACCESS CONSCIOUSNESS AND MY JOURNEY WITH LATIN DANCE

Access Consciousness has a lot of hands-on body processes that unlock trauma, upset, abuse, pain, body issues and memories from the body.

They facilitate your body and you to have a new space that is more joyful, has more ease, and a beautiful sense of connection.

Prior to Access Consciousness, although I had the practice of dance movement, I still had a lot of self-abusive thoughts and a disconnection from my body.

Now, with these body processes, I was starting to have a caring for myself that was beyond anything I had before. I could also hear my body. My body was becoming my best friend!

I was desiring more social dance so I found a social salsa night in the city. This was the beginning of me embodying the Latin dance!

It was like I was remembering something I already knew. My body just knew it. I learned so much from these Salsa nights. As a female, you have to let go of control and let the man lead.

When I would start to dance, my monkey mind would be racing! So, I would ask questions. Questions always empower you, answers disempower!

I would ask:

What would it take to be present here with me, my body and this person?

What generative energy, space and consciousness can me and my body be, to be out of control, form, structure, significance, linearity, definition, conclusion for all eternity with total ease?

I would ask my body to trust again and let go.

What would it take to lower my barriers here and receive?

Body, who would you like to dance with?

After a while of going to these events and dancing with all these different people, I realized my body didn't desire to dance with everyone! So, I asked my body to find a body that would be fun, kind and nurturing to dance with.

I met this friendly, bright, alive Columbian guy named Alex. He was a strong leader and I was able to let go with him and let him lead me in a way like no other before.

He had a kindness and caring with my body. When he touched me, my whole body melted. He didn't have any ulterior motives, just pure kindness.

Alex became one of my greatest teachers. The greatest gift was his vulnerability, which allowed me to trust him. My body healed and let go from his kindness and the joy of the dance gave me an even greater joy of living.

YOGA AND ACCESS CONSCIOUSNESS

Yoga has been a major contribution to me, my body and my life. When I first moved to America two years ago, Hot Yoga was a tool for me. It gave me the strength and stamina to create a life here.

There were so many times in the first six months where I was so challenged, and I struggled. I wanted to give up and go home.

Instead, I would show up for a Hot Yoga class, do the yoga sequence while sweating and with tears and I would leave the class transformed.

> *"Yoga does not change*
> *the way we see things,*
> *it transforms the person who sees."*
> *~ BKS Ivengar*

When I go to Yoga, I ask the Access Consciousness questions throughout the class.

First, do you realize how much people judge themselves? When you are in a class and you find yourself starting to judge yourself, for not being fit enough, or for not practicing enough, or for not being stronger, or for still having that extra weight on your belly you can ask: Who does this belong to?® and return to sender with consciousness attached.

This will create space in your world so you don't have to spend the whole class with all these judgments in your head.

Before I go to any class or do any form of movement. I ask my body:

What would be fun for you today body?

What movement will energize you today?

I don't go to Yoga classes every day. My body likes to go to Yoga some days, sometimes it asks for movement on the beach, other times it asks for movement by the pool and some days for a rest. I go with what is light for my body.

Would you be willing to be in the question every day, about what would be fun and energize your body?

NEVER GIVE UP, NEVER GIVE IN

When I was in Ireland, I had taken a Burlesque fitness course with Sarah Kelly, a powerful girl who was a fun, bright diamond.

We were women of all different sizes and shapes, and in that class I saw how these ladies started to flirt with their bodies and have fun.

Now this felt more like empowerment through dance! I so desired to create more of this when I moved to America.

This, combined with all I knew about Yoga, Ecstatic dance, Kundalini, 5 Rhythms, Access Consciousness and salsa had me flowing with many creative ideas.

*"The only way to make sense
out of change is to plunge into it,
move with it, and join the dance."
~ Alan Watts*

I embraced everything I knew and created Shine Movements. I started with Shine Movements classes on Delray Beach in the early morning sun.

Every class is different. There is no structure. The class moves from Yoga to Burlesque to flowing dance, to Kundalini breath work, to Access Consciousness questions and clearings, to Latin moves, to out of control, out of structure dance, to ease and expansion exercises, to melting into the ground.

Every class is different according to who comes to the class and what they are asking for.

There have been so many times where I wanted to quit and give up. What I am doing is different and outside the box.

As my beautiful friend Patty Alfonso says, "What we are doing is different. We have created a new reality with bodies, dance and movement. It may take people a while to catch on..."

All it takes is one person coming to my class and when I see the transformation that happens - the person becomes more joyful, they start creating their dreams or they find loving relationships - that's all I need to keep going.

Do not ever quit. Never give in. Never give up. Continue going and creating.

Shine Movements has grown and is now offered at various locations and for different age levels. I also created 'Body Flirt'. An easy to follow, burlesque inspired dance movement class with props, designed to empower women to flirt, play and embrace their bodies while also getting fit.

Leave your judgments at the door and fall in love with your body. Be its best friend!

And there is SO much more to come. I'm only getting started. I have only just begun.

My last line to you is this: Do not ever give up on your dreams. Even if nobody else gets it. Follow what you know. You are unique and you have something special to gift this world that nobody else does. Keep going. Keep moving.

"Never give up on what you really want to do. The person with big dreams is more powerful than the person with all the facts."
~ Albert Einstein

Amy Shine

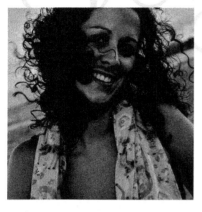

Amy Shine is an Access Consciousness Certified Bars & Body Facilitator®, Dance Movement Facilitator, Thai Yoga Vedic Massage Therapist and the creator of Shine Movements.

Amy grew up in Ireland where she received a Bachelor of Arts Degree in Social Care. Amy's own personal journey includes various healing modalities.

Amy works with children and teenagers doing Yoga, Dance and energy therapy. She also teaches free flowing, transformational movement classes for adults that combine Yoga, Kundalini breath work, all forms of dance, Access Consciousness and more.

If you'd like to learn more about Amy, you can find her online in social media and at:

www.ShineMovements.com
ww.amyshine.accessconsciousness.com

Chapter 5

Delicious Dance
By Rachael O'Brien

And I said to my body softly,
"I want to be your friend."
It took a long breath and replied,
"I have been waiting for you."

I was born to be a leader. Sometimes leadership looks a lot different than what you think its going look like. I am not a professional dancer nor do I dance with the grace and flexibility like some of the dancers in this world.

What I do know is that dance has no form, no structure, no significance and zero judgment of me or my body. For me dance is beyond all of that.

Dance is like Rumi's quote: "Out beyond ideas of wrong and right, there is a field, where I dance, I'll meet you there."

It's pretty amazing and quite hilarious for me to acknowledge that it has been a dream of mine to write a book for many years, and if you told me that my first book would be a collaboration about dance I would have laughed my ass off.

Isn't it amazing how things never show up the way you think they will? What a beautiful way to start, to be part of a collaboration and to talk about something I love, not as a professional dance teacher, but as someone who always knew the gift of delicious dance to my life and my body.

So my journey with delicious dance started as a very young girl in Ireland, and it began with a traditional form of dance called Irish Dancing.

I absolutely loved it! There were no "Beyonce's" back then. No twerking. To dance sexually would have been a mortal sin (a Catholic saying, that you will burn in hell because you are so bad).

So as a beautiful little girl I started to dance. In Ireland we learn our 1,2,3s and then 1,2,3,4,5,6,7, and 1,2,3,3,4,5,6,7. It's fast, it moves quick and some of it looks like tap dancing. Think river dance.

So I am three years of age, and my favorite thing in the world is to have a red ribbon in my hair and Irish dance. Dance has always been a space of fun, movement and potency for me.

It was never a problem, steps were never a problem, just listen to the beat and follow it. I have never learned a step of a dance through watching someone do it slowly. It doesn't work like that for me.

I watch the person move and listen to the beat and play with it. It fascinates me, how bodies move... to watch and see the capacities the body has to play and mimic.

I loved to be the best at everything. It was fun for me! Of course, this inspiration only came when I actually liked something. If I didn't like it, I was usually crap at it.

Anything I have ever liked in life, I have had an ability to learn very fast. That's just the way it is for me.

When it came to Irish dancing, I went to school at age four

and entered into every competition I could. I had a plaque with one hundred medals by the time I was six.

My mother adored it. She was a seamstress so she would make ribbons for my hair. I loved the snow white bobby socks we would wear with the black soft dancing shoes wrapped around the socks.

Then something changed. When I reached seven years old, it got very competitive and it wasn't fun for me anymore. The judges picked their favorites or girls who wore the best dresses and that didn't work for me.

I would see a gorgeous dancer not win but a girl with a magnificent uniform or an aunt as a judge would. That was the end of competitions for me. I have this tendency to do something that I like, learn it fast, and then if there is a part of it I don't like I just lose interest super fast. It's so funny for me to realize while writing this, how I function!

Backstage at a competition I just decided I am done with this. Irish dance didn't stop there, I always dance, if I am at a party and Irish music comes on I will dance.

Looking back, my love of movement has been something personal to me. It's not something that can be judgeable by anyone else. Even at the age of seven the competition and judges didn't make sense to me.

I adore music, just adore it! As a teenager I would dance in the street. When Michael Jackson released *Thriller* I was going to modern dance. I remember all of the girls in the park and my best friend Raymond learning all the moves. Having a big ghetto blaster and dancing for hours until we all got the moves. We made Raymond be Michael turning into the Wolf, it was so funny.

I loved the way Michael followed Ola Ray in the video. The way he walked beside her while she pretends to ignore him and by his persistence to dance she starts to smile and he seduces her through dance.

It is just gorgeous, how bodies get happy in dance and any problems you have just fade away. One thing I know about me if there is even the tiniest possibility to be joyous I will choose it.

"Cause this is thriller, thriller night..." Sing it with me!!

When I look at dance, it has been the gift that has allowed my kids and I to have fun together. My 23 year old daughter is gifted in movement and, wow, can she move her body! My kids have always danced, they love parties, they love music.

I was a huge Cure fan as a teenager and would play the music while cleaning my house. One night my eldest daughter disappeared from our lounge and came back with the younger one dressed up as cats and dancing around the room.

When it comes to business, I don't teach dance. I teach movement. Conscious Movement. I am a trained Pilates teacher and just love facilitating people to have more presence and awareness with their body.

It still blows my mind how the body's capacity to stretch and relax in movement is supported massively in a space of no judgment.

People have so many points of view around a movement or dance being performed correctly. This to me is total exclusion and I open the door to anyone who would like to move no matter what their age and size. I know this is the reason people have chosen to work with me for years.

MY JOURNEY WITH ACCESS CONSCIOUSNESS®

I like to keep things really simple.

Let's look at the little girl with the golden hair and the tanned, chunky gorgeous thighs who loved to dance and joy was always the choice of the day...

All of a sudden, I am 40 and I have no clue where the joy went. I am living a super stressed life as a mother of three and reached breaking point. Life became about paying bills, and being resentful for how often I was working.

Do you ever ask yourself these questions?

Where am I? What's fun for me? And then genuinely not remember what you were like as a kid?

I have done many healing modalities and one of them was *"A Course in Miracles"*. I loved that book dearly, I hear people say its difficult to understand. I didn't have that, I totally got what it was about and really knew somewhere that a miracle was a shift in perception.

While going through that book, for my life, I was asking to be the gift they said I could be in the book.

Everywhere in the book it said all things were possible. I certainly knew that on an energetic level but not in my day to day life.

I knew there was another way to live, a way of joy and possibility. My life was repetitive. I was not in a good place financially and my relationship with my partner wasn't fun. We stayed in, paid the bills and looked after our kids. I got depressed.

When you know life can be a gift, it gets super heavy when you are not living that way. *"A Course in Miracles"* talks about finding your own internal teacher. I know this book created the demand in my world.

Through doing the course I recognized I had a lot of programming about life being tough, a lot of lack with money and a lot of thoughts that didn't create ease in my life.

One day, after reading the book I went out to my back garden. I sat in shell stretch and begged the Earth to bring me processes that could unlock all the fear programs in my body. I am getting chills writing this now.

The very next day, my sister who I have so much gratitude for, rang me and said she had talked to a friend in North Carolina who told her about Access Consciousness®.

My sister has lived in the US for 17 years now and was at home for a few months. She told me there was an Access Consciousness Certified Facilitator coming to the Cork Mind, Body and Spirit Conference. She said: "and I have no idea why I am telling you this, I really think you should be there." So I went.

Now the piece I would like to tell you is that I had a really heavy period that day, my head was racing, my body was like someone had rolled over me in a truck. My face was old and stressed, but I got up and went.

I have been gifted with a super open mind. I am the type of person that will always check something out. If it worked great, if it didn't I would move on, sometimes a bit battered.

So I go to the Cork Mind, Body and Spirit Conference and I hear the first talk about money. She asked: "If money was standing in front of you would it come hang out with you or would it back away?"

I walked out of there, nodding my head. The information

given to me just made sense, I had never seen a message so clearly delivered through tools and words. Then I got this energy therapy called The Access Bars® run on my body. They said it relaxes the body and helps with mind chatter.

While getting my bars run, this little girl about seven years old stood next to the bed. It was so weird for me as I saw myself at that age and how beautiful I was.

I had been abused as a child and didn't really know how to deal with it. The memories got more active when I had my kids and, at this stage, my body was really showing me what it wanted to get rid of.

I had a lot of unresolved sadness with the abuse and knew I no longer wanted to perpetuate that fear on my kids. I was paranoid over them and had a lot of control.

I would also get these anger bursts where I would want to break everything in the house. I couldn't control them and would want to kill myself with the guilt and shame of what I had done in front of my kids afterwards. I now know the worst thing for me in my life is to see my kids terrified when I would explode.

Because this little girl contributed a commitment to me to change these behaviors no matter what, I can truly say today the Access Consciousness tools have changed my life.

I now live in control of my life. If anger comes in, I know it is an energy that stops me being present and I know how to deal with it.

The greatest information I ever received is that anger is a lie you have bought about you. If ever you get angry ask yourself:

What's the lie spoken and unspoken?

In Access Consciousness, we call anger a distractor implant. In other words, it stops YOU from being you.

That night I walked out of the Cork City Hall different. I wasn't sure how I was different but I *knew* it.

The river of the city looked different, I heard the bird's wings flap as they flew, the world looked beautiful to me.

Einstein once asked: "Is the world a friendly place? He suggested this was a question you had to ask yourself to see if you were functioning from fear or love.

In truth, before this day, the world wasn't a friendly place for me. I had moments of bliss, moments of joy, moments of being stunned by the beauty of my kids, moments of being blown away by the beauty of the planet while sitting in Dzogchen Beara, a Buddhist retreat center in West Cork, Ireland.

The problem was I would have this in a workshop and then return to my life as a working mum and I would lose it.

The festival in Cork was for three days so of course I went back the next day and stayed there all day. I got my Access Bars run again and felt better. I went back the third day and felt way better and lighter.

I said to the Facilitator: "If you think I am stalking you I am!" She responded: "I would too if I was you, I am pretty awesome."

She had gifted me the energy of my favorite quote in the book, "*Return to Love*" by Marianne Williamson:

"Our deepest fear is not that we are inadequate. Our deepest fear is that we are powerful beyond measure. It is our light, not our darkness that most frightens us.

We ask ourselves, 'Who am I to be brilliant, gorgeous,

talented, fabulous?' Actually, who are you not to be? You are a child of God. Your playing small does not serve the world. There is nothing enlightened about shrinking so that other people won't feel insecure around you. We are all meant to shine, as children do. We were born to make manifest the glory of God that is within us. It's not just in some of us; it's in everyone. And as we let our own light shine, we unconsciously give other people permission to do the same. As we are liberated from our own fear, our presence automatically liberates others."

I found out there was a training in The Bars on in Dublin followed by a 4 day Foundation and Level 1 class.

I also found out the classes cost about 1100 Euro. I went home and spoke to my husband Derek and said: "Der, I have to go here."

He knew when I had to go do something. He said: "Go for it and we will figure the money out later." So I went to Dublin. My sister couldn't believe it.

I stayed with my friend Aoife. What a support she was to me that weekend! I left Dublin different. Again I wasn't sure in what way, I just knew I was.

FEAR IN MY BODY

Now this piece I have to tell you. I had a fear in my body when a guy would approach me from behind. I would freeze.

MTVSS is an Access Body Process to help your body function with ease. After the first time I had it run, my friend Pat came up behind me and threw me up in the air, I started giggling like a little kid.

When my mind caught up with what had just happened I

knew my body had let go of that "fear" point of view. I had also suffered from Post Traumatic Shock Seizures and I had the last one ever at my first Foundation Class.

I chose then and there to facilitate this work. I knew a different reality was available to anyone who sought it. I chose to train in the Access Bars, and go on to train as a Certified Facilitator.

The day I left Dublin I had 50 Euro in my joint bank account with Derek. He rang me while I was driving home to tell me we had received a tax rebate of 1450 Euro. It was roughly the amount it had cost me to be in Dublin. Thank you Universe! Thank you to Derek for filling out forms to check our taxes!

About the same time as Foundation I had started to dance again, I was doing a lot of five rhythms dancing. I enjoyed being in a space of no alcohol and a space to dance the way I like to dance. I am pretty crazy when I dance sometimes and super funny.

I loved that it was a place where you could move the way your body wished to. In Ireland dancing is really only available in nightclubs where people are drunk and messy. The other alternative is to go to a structured class. I knew at this stage in my life neither worked for me.

SKIP AHEAD 10 MONTHS AND I MET THIS AMAZING GIRL CALLED AMY SHINE.

I had gone into Alcoholics Anonymous as a last resort about two years before The Foundation Class. I told them I hadn't been drinking but I was suicidal. I used to drink as a teen and maybe I was an alcoholic so they said give it a whirl.

I actually liked it there at the start. I met super kind

people in AA and I also had so much fun. The stories in an AA room are absolutely hilarious and people give them no significance whatsoever.

This girl caught my eye, Amy Shine, I just loved her when I met her. We became friends quickly I told her about Access Consciousness and she did an Access Bars class with me in January 2013.

Amy chose to do her thesis on dance, so we started a dance class in my studio. We had so much fun there. We laughed we cried, we screamed, we jumped, we sweat.

This studio became the place for me to dance. My kids danced in that room more times than I can mention. Birthday parties were held in that room and many a kid came to a dance party that turned into a sleepover there. I am sure many a kid will have a memory of that room.

In Access Consciousness, we talk about being you and changing the world. I know people get so happy when I dance. My business has expanded due to me talking openly and truthfully about my body. How it likes to move. How I love to be sensual whether it be through dance or touch.

When you come alive and dance, everyone wants to come play with you. I asked my man today what would he say about me and dance and he said: "You are totally alive. It's so inviting its impossible not to join you."

And my kids they just laugh their ass off at me when I am dancing to Jesus Walks by Kanye. That's my inspirational song.

"Buyacka Ha, kick ass Zeena Warrior"

I have just created a new Specialty Class in Access Consciousness called: So you think you can't dance?

The class is about stepping into the five elements of intimacy, which are: Honor, Trust, Allowance, Vulnerability, and Gratitude through movement with your body. It's inviting you to a new possibility with your body.

Today, I am living the dream while I am awake. I get to facilitate people from all over the globe. I am creating a global transformational business.

Did I ever think this was possible four and a half years ago? The truth is: no. So often I ask clients:

What have you judged as impossible in your life that if you were willing to receive the possibility of it, would open the door to actualizing it?

Usually their heads spin for a while and then they get the awareness of how much they are refusing to receive based on a judgment they decided on. Usually the judgments are: "I could never have that... that's too much, so why would I even ask for it."

I know today when you are willing to be you, speak honestly, dance on the street to a busker, and really be you no matter what, it opens a space in someone's world for them to have fun and be them.

What a gift to facilitate people to choose beyond limitations in their life!

My Favourite Tool

The tools and processes in Access Consciousness have changed everything in my life that's not working. This body of work has given me back the child within me.

Today I went to Galway with my gorgeous man, I danced on the street to a guy playing the saxophone, then in the city a busker was singing the tune from Grease: "You're the one that I want..."and instantly I started dancing and singing to my man.

I have gorgeous movement with my body and it shows me what is fun for it. Today I went for breakfast and I wasn't sure if I would like to eat, so I went outside and said: "Body what would you like to eat?"

I sat beside a woman and we started to chat. She was eating strawberries, banana, berries, kiwi with yoghurt and honey. That was exactly what I was looking for!

How cool is it to have conscious communion with your body?!

While writing this chapter, I have opened up to receiving so much gratitude for the body of work called Access Consciousness.

Most of all I am receiving me and my capacity to create my life in a way that works for me. I actually changed a lot of crap in my life and...what else is truly possible?

I am super excited to be alive. Yesterday I woke and was singing and dancing receiving the possibility of having my life as the gift it is meant to be.

Did I really know cognitively that was possible? Did I know energetically? Yes!

What if life is a gift? How would you choose to create your life if you knew you could not fail?

I have really looked and reflected at where I was four and a half years ago and where I am now. It's incredible to acknowledge the change in my life, with my body, my relationships, my finances, my day to day living, my creation, my friends and most of all my relationship with me.

I like me! I am this gorgeous collection of awesomeness, totally undefined. I adore me, who I be and what I choose to create in the world.

Now I would like to share my favourite tool. I adore them all but the one that wins hands down is:

"Who does this belong to?

Return to sender with consciousness attached"

Okay, why, you may ask, is this my favourite tool?

Great question!

In Access Consciousness, we talk about how 99 percent of our thoughts, ideas, beliefs and emotions are not ours. 99 percent of that monkey mind isn't even yours!!

I hear you say: "OK, great concept."

What if I told you that all the places your life doesn't work for you is where you bought someone else's thought, idea, belief, point of view about how you have to do life.

Why do we say return to sender with consciousness attached? Right now, its seems like just a concept. Here is the magic piece... if you actually start to use this, you will get a level of freedom you never knew possible.

You will become aware of all the places that you bought someone else's version of life. You buy it, take it home and eat it. Mmm not my best choice and maybe not yours either.

What if you became aware of everything you bought, returned what didn't work for you and used what did work for you?

Then you would have total choice.

This tool is not a concept. This tool is like the book *The Never Ending Story*. You start to know that life can be created from ease, joy and glory.

This Who does it belong to? ™ tool, don't take my word for it. Do your own experiment. Access Consciousness has created a FREE app to help you! Check it out if you if you have an Android or iPhone. You can download the app and set reminders!

I was at a party in Copenhagen. I was super happy and dancing, having a wonderful time, and then I got hit with this weird feeling of sadness. I got a ping in my pocket, I took out my phone there was my reminder, Who does this belong to? Return to sender with consciousness attached.

Guess what?! It wasn't mine!

It lightened up straight away. If it lightens up it's not yours. You gotta get that you are aware, you are so aware! You pick up on a feeling, you think its yours without even questioning it and the reality is it's not.

It could be the person next to you at the party, the fact you are aware of it, means it's actually not you. How cool is that?!

My suggestion is you play with it, and let it work in your life. Please do let me know if it creates space and ease for you. I really think we should have been given this tool at birth.

Ask yourself: "As a little kid, were you ever sad or did you *pretend* to be sad so you fit in?"

Chances are you were super happy. That's the true you. Have fun playing with this tool!

So thank you for reading my chapter I hoped it has

contributed to you in some way. Here are some questions you can play with:

If you were trusting you what would you choose?

What if you saw you as the gift of possibility this world has been waiting for?

What would you like to create our world as?

What else is possible beyond anything we have ever known?

Thank you again for the gift you be.

~ Rachael

Rachael O'Brien

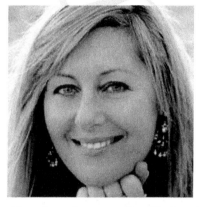

Rachael O'Brien, CFMW, is a Transformational Life Coach, Access Consciousness® Certified Facilitator, radio show host and mother of three children aged 16, 17 and 22.

She travels the world empowering people to create ease in their lives and allowing them to finally be themselves. Rachael is known for her exuberance and infectious joy.

Raised in Cork, Ireland, Rachael struggled in school. By the age of fourteen she was drinking alcohol. After battling numerous health issues and trying all sorts of different modalities for change, she began to ask for something greater. Then Access Consciousness showed up in her life. Using these amazing tools, Rachael has been able to change her relationships, finances, and body.

Today Rachael works privately with several of the top business leaders, entrepreneurs and philanthropists in Europe.

You can contact Rachael at: www.rachaelobrien.org

You can also find her on YouTube and Facebook

Chapter 6

Dancing as the Creation of Greater Possibilities
By Kalpana Raghuraman

When Access Consciousness® came into my life, I was way into my career as a dancer and choreographer.

I would say dance was in my life ever since I was in my mother's womb - my mom was one of Netherlands' first Indian dance teachers and was very actively teaching and performing while she was pregnant with me.

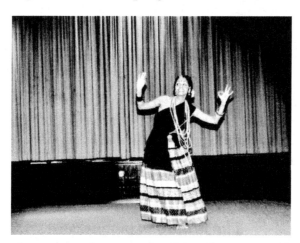

She ran her own dance school and was teaching and performing, so my body was used to having moving, dancing bodies around me.

I learnt many movements just by watching her, and watching her teach. There is no cognition of it, my body seems to have just duplicated it and tapped into her and the other bodies around me, to get the information.

What can your body tap into now that would allow it to access the information that is required to move in ways that would be fun and expansive?!

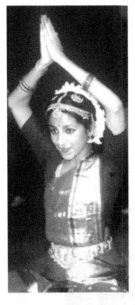

I was very young myself when I took the stage dancing, speaking and singing.

When I look back at it now, there was no significance for me in that at all. Dancing was just one of the many things I did.

By the age of five, I was performing on stage as if it was the most normal thing to do, just like breathing... and I guess it was!

What was total ease for you as a kid that you turned off since others did not have or choose that capacity?

What was so natural and ease for you and your body at a young age that you have not acknowledged, that if you would - would allow you to tap into that again...and have it available to you at your mere request?!

Empowering dancers with Access Consciousness® tools: The Malay experience

The cool thing with Access Consciousness tools is that I was immediately able to apply these tools to what I was creating in the studio.

I remember two weeks after my first Access Bars® class,

I went to Malaysia to create a performance. I had been invited to select dancers from a dance company and create a performance for them.

And it was without even a single thought that I immediately started using the tools in the process:

Asking questions

Clearing the places and spaces where they were judging themselves and hence limiting what was possible

Empowering them to function from their strengths and what was fun for them

The effect was astounding to say the least. Dancers blossomed in front of my very eyes.

I remember one dancer who seemed invisible during the workshop week. I knew there was more to this obedient quiet girl than met the eye. By the end of the creation period and by the time she was on stage, she was a roaring, strong presence.

Audience members that had been seeing her on stage for years could not believe their eyes, and told me it was as if for the very first time, they finally saw her for who she really is.

In Indian dance, as in many classical dance forms, we are taught totally from the idea of 'disciplining' the body and mind. There is a lot of force, a lot of push and not much kindness.

I however have always functioned from acknowledging dancers for their talents and capacities. My mother had shown me the possibilities that are available if you are present with what is true for each body instead of functioning from the 'shoulds'.

So I did not do what they were used to –

I did not create distance through authority

I did not discipline them by insulting them

I did not judge them

I did not compare them to others

Instead...

I was ME.

I was my silly, funny me, making my dirty jokes and having way more fun than a person is allowed to when in the serious process of creating art.

I was just ME.

I invited them to be themselves.

I invited them to allow their bodies to show us what was possible.

In that way I showed them another way of creating and another way to be with moving bodies.

> *What does your body know*
> *that only your body knows?*

> *What possibility can your body*
> *show you and the world*
> *that you have not yet considered?*

These dancers were awestruck.

In the last week of a five-week creation period, one of the dancers asked me – did you notice our faces in the first few days?

"You actually asked US what we thought of certain things! You asked our point of view and there was space to voice what we had as perspectives and ideas."

I had chosen the theme of Superheroes of Indian mythology, and in fact the theme helped them to look at themselves in a totally different way.

I had asked each of the dancers to pick a personality from Indian mythology that they felt inspired by or somehow connected to.

Allowing them to actually let their bodies tap into what qualities these superheroes had, allowed them to move from a whole different space than they had up to then.

Empowering people to know that they know through dance!

DEFINITION IS A LIMITATION

About a year before I found the tools of Access Consciousness, I started to dance less and choreograph more.

I became aware of how many ideas I had that I wanted to put together. Not being on stage myself, allowed me to see all the segments and enjoy the orchestration of a performance including light, set-design, costume and music.

As I started to dance less, I started to see myself more as a 'choreographer' which of course was a total limitation.

When I started to play with the Access Consciousness tools and started to ask more questions – I realized that by defining myself as a choreographer now, I was limiting what I could create and what my body could contribute.

What definition of you are you using to limit the contribution your body can be are you choosing?

As soon as I became aware of how my decision and definition of being a choreographer was limiting me, my body was immediately able to be more of a contribution to the dancers I was working with.

And not only that, also to the people around me.

Just because I was dancing less, did not mean my body would stop the joy of moving, or stop moving other bodies!

What movement does your body inspire in others that you have never considered and not yet acknowledged?

Now when I choreograph, I am so aware of how my body informs other bodies. And that my body shows other bodies what is possible. The same thing occurs when I am facilitating Access Consciousness classes.

In turn, these bodies start to move in ways that are different, allowing for so much more than seemed possible before.

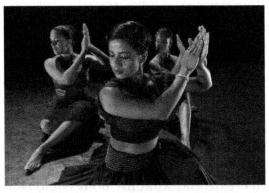

Kandam Ostinato photo by Robert Benschop

MY DANCE COMPANY

When I started with Access Consciousness I was a freelance artist. I was an affiliate choreographer in one of the largest production houses of contemporary dance in the Netherlands.

My time there was extremely fruitful. Using the tools, and moving at the speed of space, I was able to create a lot. I was ready to fly off, leave the bounds of the known and the established, to create my own dance company. Which I did!

My company received funding for two years by the city, allowing my dance company to be one of the first Indian contemporary dance companies to be recognized as part of the mainstream art scene.

Three of my company dancers have also been introduced to Access Consciousness. They have all learned the Access Bars® and have taken The Foundation class with me as well as plenty of other classes.

We use the tools all the time when we are creating. We use clearings to get out of judgments and limitations, we use verbal processing to step into greater possibilities and we use body processes to support the bodies, to strengthen them and also to heal them when injured or sore.

It has been one of my dreams ever since I started Access Consciousness to have dancers I work with actually use these tools.

It is no longer a dream – I have created it! And wow what an amazing gift. For me, for them and for the performances we are creating.

BEYOND THE LIES

The topics that come up with Access Consciousness have also been a strong inspiration for me and my dance creations. They continue to inspire new works.

We unlock lies and limitations in Access Consciousness by looking at our points of view. The tools have made everything more succinct, more effective, so much more creative and generative and with total ease.

For many years, I have been looking at the essence of Indian dance forms by peeling off all the form, structure and significance.

By unlocking these codes, these solidifications and limitations, I have been creating a whole new language of movement and aesthetics, really taking off layers of restrictions on a physical, choreographic level.

What becomes available is so much information, inspiration and beauty.

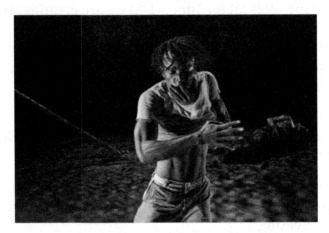

'Towards Dawn', photo by Robert Benschop

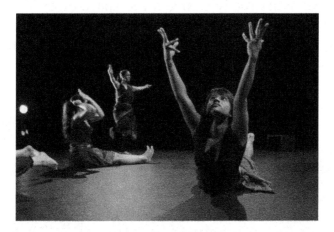

'Through the eyes of my city', photo by Robert Benschop

I have also been infusing insights from Access Consciousness into the creation of the work itself. So besides applying it to the creation process as described in the Malaysian example, also with the topics and awareness.

Tightrope Walker for example is all about shame and self-judgment. Topics we look at so much in Access Consciousness and for me to see how these things also affect the body and how it moves has been truly a life changing experience.

In *Tightrope Walker* I used the points of view that the solo dancer had taken over and bought from others such as 'you will never do it right'. We gave a voice to these points of view through movements.

These movements in turn allowed the dancer to release these points of view and allowed the audience to receive the shift of this, unlocking the lies around bodies, moving and being through dance.

I can say that the acoustical vibrations of the music and

the movements really changed the space every time this particular solo was performed. It moved and shifted things *within* people. The audience always left different from how they arrived.

'Tightrope Walker'; photo by Robert Benschop

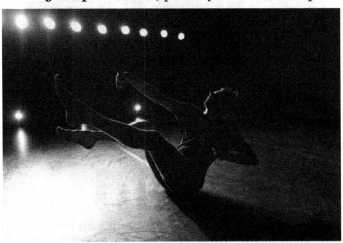

What acoustical vibration can you always be with your body that would allow people to shift and transform by being in your presence?

MYSELF AS A DANCER

I have been trained in the classical Indian dance form Bharatanatyam. Like many classical forms, this form is extremely rich and is simultaneously passed on with a whole set of judgments and restrictions.

I used to always get angry at this and it was one of the reasons I started to create my own work. So that I did not have to perpetrate and perpetuate these lies and limitations that did not make any sense to me.

These Access Consciousness tools work and since I always was aware of these things not being true – it was a huge relief to no longer make them relevant and function from my knowing and awareness!

What do you know about moving that has been sold as a lie in order to restrict and limit people?

Bharatanatyam performance in India

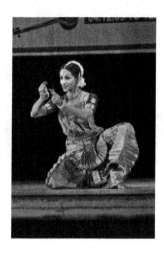

Since I have been using the Access Consciousness tools, I have become aware of how differently I am moving when I dance.

There is so much more ease and fun. And, it is more from a space of choice and knowing instead of from a space of judgment, and figuring it out. How does it get any better?!

Really including my body consciously helped this a lot.

Body what do you know here?
What do you require here?

These are simple questions to start opening the gates to

the knowledge of our bodies.

So what questions could you ask your body to gain access to its infinite knowing?!

'**The spirit of Frida**' ; photo by Robert Benschop

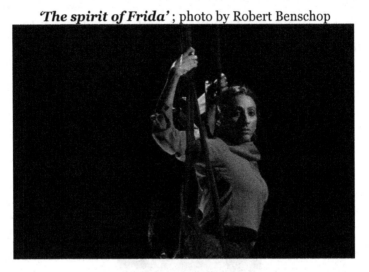

ACCESS THE JOY OF MOVEMENT

In 2015 I had created a specialty class around bodies and their energies called Seduction of Embodiment.   I knew there was something else that was also asking to be created.

Aware that my capacity with moving bodies could also be a contribution beyond the dance field, I spoke to Gary Douglas about what I could create with the Access Consciousness tools as a specialty class.

He immediately said "You have so much ease with your body and with moving. You also have such a clear strong capacity to be in communion with other bodies and show them what is possible. Call it Joy of Movement and build that as your class".

At first I was like:

Joy of Movement?! Really?!

I thought it would be boring and dull and I totally dismissed this brilliant man and his brilliant awareness.

A few months later I woke up:

JOY OF MOVEMENT, YES!

I finally became aware of what I could create with this class and what Gary Douglas was showing me as a possibility.

I became more aware of all the bodies that desire to move–

Move without being judged

Move without any limitations

Move without having to be creating 'something'

So I developed a class where we clear what points of view we took over about moving bodies so that we can tap into what our own body knows and start having fun from there.

What way does your body desire to move that you have not even considered?

Aware of the fact that bodies would desire to move during this class, I worked together with the Italian music composer Simone Giacomini, who composed for many of my contemporary dance works.

He composed music for the exercises that we do during the class – each exercise is accompanied by music that allows the body to tap into that vibration through this music -- and what I have seen occur is simply awesome and magic.

I was able to see change for bodies that were so stuck, so judged, people who were feeling so uncomfortable, so contracted. They all started to relax, to become present, to melt and to move from a space of joy and ease!

What ease and joy is possible for you and your body that

seems impossible now?

And now, besides the dance performances that I create and tour, I also facilitate these classes all over the world.

The space it has been opening up for people is such a gift.

No separation

More than ever am I aware of how dancing has been so separate from daily life.

My mother-in-law, who is from Burkina Faso, always responds to good news by...dancing!

We celebrate life through dance and yet there is so much judgment on this.

What if that no longer has to be true?!

For me, I can see how the more aware I am becoming, the more I can receive dance and movement as the gift of living.

What if we can include our bodies - our moving, wise and joyful bodies in every aspect of living?

I am so grateful that I have the gift of creating dance and facilitating dance as a way to open up the space for more.

What invitation can this be for you - To walk, skip, dance at the rhythm of your body's joy?!

Kalpana Raghuraman

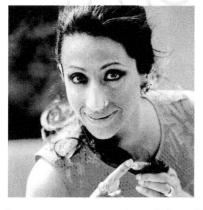

Kalpana Raghuraman is an Access Consciousness® Certified Facilitator and artistic director of her own dance company: St. Kalpana – Arts Reimagined.

Kalpana travels the world creating change through her facilitation and her dance creations. She facilitates her own Access Specialty classes: Joy of Movement and Seduction of Embodiment. She also facilitates Joy of Business, Being You, Right Voice for You and Talk to the Entities.

Kalpana's love for and ease with bodies allows her to include her body when facilitating and invites others to including their bodies more.

Her sharpness, humor and kindness make her a sought-after facilitator and choreographer.

For more information about Kalpana visit:

www.kalpanaraghuraman.com

Chapter 7

Dance with Me
By Monica Mata Gilliam

What is it, I wonder, that you call dancing?

Is dancing what all those sweaty bodies are doing in nightclubs and living rooms around the world?

Does it require music? Or training?

Would you call yourself a dancer? Or, is dancing somehow limited to those often suffering performers who devote their lives to high art and poverty?

Oh please, no!

Look at the world around you. Where is the dancing there? Time and again, the poets of the world have gifted us their perspectives on dance. Their words have wandered around the world and taken root in our imaginations.

I would be surprised, if at some point, you have not heard about the dancing of the leaves or the light or the water. What is it that transforms the movements of the world into a dance? Do we, perhaps, simply call something a dance when we take a moment to appreciate it?

That is, of course, a leading question. It is my present hypothesis and one that I would gladly instill within you if you would be so kind as to allow me that honor.

And, while I've got your attention and you are sitting there, generously reading my thoughts, would you be willing to put aside the notions of dance you have been carrying and follow me into a swirling, winding exploration of dance?

Would you allow these words to awaken all that is possible for conscious embodiment with, through and beyond your body?

Here is the framework that I offer for our journey: at its very root, dance is *PRESENCE*. It is the exuberantly shifting and interesting points of view that each of us can choose whenever or wherever we'd like.

To dance is to consciously perceive and play with all that we are aware of. Your relative level of awareness doesn't really matter. The only requirement is that you give yourself the freedom to move. And, oh, there is so much you can move!

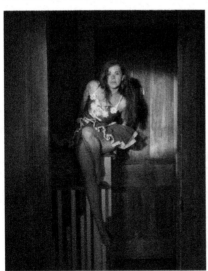

Photo by: Bobby Bonsey

The life-changing magic of dance must not be underestimated. The presence of your consciousness through your body and your being offers a dynamic means to facilitate change in all areas of your life (and the world) with greater ease than you might imagine.

That playful, dancing presence of your consciousness communing with the world around you can open new doorways into the delights of this physical existence we are presently embodying.

Dancing, as viewed through this lens, becomes an incredibly potent, transformative act.

Throughout my life, I have had the pleasure to dance my way through many seemingly tricky situations. More recently, dancing through the wild fields of energy I am immersed in, has led me to working with others.

Presence and movement have been my secret weapons as I have coached, prodded, teased, and challenged the fellow seekers of the world to step out of their personal prisons and into the creation of the lives they know are possible.

I am enormously grateful for the gifts of insight and awareness that my body, my countless teachers and this great earth have facilitated within me.

Allow me to share with you a bit of my story and how I came to dance with the world in the ways that I now do.

I rode horses when I was younger. There was nothing quite so wonderful as flying along, jumping over logs and hedges with an enormously powerful creature as my friend and transport. What a dreamy, fortunate time that was!?!

And then, high school happened.

Though my body had been wildly shifting since my conception, suddenly its changes were being given a different kind of attention.

My friends, family, and even strangers began to direct different types of energies at me. Everything was steeped in greater **significance**, but nobody was being very clear about ways to navigate all of that.

The best I could ascertain was that I was walking along the edge of a very dangerous, possibly harmful world and that my body had a great deal to do with that danger.

The joys of wildly galloping around quickly transformed as body shame and confusion were projected at me from all sides. Hanging out at the barn became less and less of a priority until one day my horse was sold and I was left to figure out what to do with myself.

I tried TV for a while.

I watched hours of sitcoms back-to-back as I waited, bored, for some adventure or other to present itself. Unfortunately, the suburbs of San Antonio, Texas did not provide the inspiration I was seeking; and so, TV it was.

I remember lying on my parents' bed in their dark room, watching a tiny little screen. Each afternoon after school I'd fill my head with countless teen-based dramas.

Uncertain of what to do with the changes in my body and my high school world, I'd dive into the imagined, pointless controversies of pretend high school students.

What a strange ride that was!

I had always been a sensitive kid, acutely aware of the emotional ups and downs of those around me. Watching the awkward situations these fictional characters encountered was excruciating! I'd sit there, concerned and embarrassed by the very plot twists that kept me from just turning the damn shows off!

My almost overwhelming concern for everyone's wellbeing left my spirit in a sort of "empathic distress" and my body in knots.

You should have seen me squirming around the room with my eyes glued to the screen. As each show ended, I took momentary stock of my body before the next show began.

More often than not, I'd find that I had twisted around

completely so that I was watching everything upside down. Or else, I'd be lying on the floor next to the bed with my feet up on the TV.

I thought it was funny how I'd end up in so many crazy positions without being aware of it. Now I realize that my body was simply responding to the energies of those shows.

All thoughts, feelings, and emotions are energies that have qualities of movement—or lack of movement—to them.

Traditional Chinese Medicine ascribes specific directions to emotions and considers the impact of energies on the body and being.

In this system, for example, anger is perceived to have an upward moving direction, whereas joy moves outward, and depression moves downward and inward.

Do any of these directions match your life experiences?

What movements and qualities have you perceived with the energy of emotions?

Have you ever wondered at the sense of flow—or lack thereof—that different energies inspire?

I greatly appreciate the awareness that Chinese Medicine's link between movement and emotion has sparked in me.

The more I explore my awareness of the ways in which energy moves, the more I recognize the vast complexity and range of energies that exist in the universe!!

Here's a little secret for you: ***no energy is good or bad.***

Each energy simply is what it is. I know, I know, on the surface this hardly seems like news. Let's go ahead and dive deeper by asking a few questions.

What is your sense of energy?

Are you willing to receive any and all energy? Or are there some energies that you have decided are best to avoid?

Are the energies that you are willing to receive "better" than the energies you are not willing to receive? Who says? Is that true all the time?

What if your judgments about energies are simply the byproduct of conclusions you have made or bought from someone else?

In this world we are indoctrinated into the judgment preferences of our family, friends, and culture. These preferences are the points of view we take about any subject, thought, action, emotion, or whatever!

We use our points of view to justify the judgments we choose to hold. And so the cycle goes on.

We have become addicted to judging everything.

I find it interesting just how often parents are given the assignment of teaching their children "right from wrong." As though anyone could ever relay enough information to stand in for someone else's awareness!

What if, instead, we could encourage each other to be aware of energy, to recognize it for what it is without judging it, and to consciously play with all of it?

What else might be possible in the world if people could be so present with all that is?

I wonder how much more ease might be available as we

seek to shift heaviness into lightness and lightness into heaviness for the sheer joy of taking part in the grand creations in which we are all involved?

What could you be aware of in each moment that might enable you to shift and change anything that is discordant into something smoother and more harmonious?

What energies do you tend to use to shift and shape your world? How are those working for you? What if you could open up greater possibilities simply by dropping the judgments that may be limiting your awareness?

I find it easiest to use body-based language to appreciate the quality and variety of different energies. For now, let's allow our palates to guide our discussion of energies.

Some energies might be described as salty and some as sweet, while others may be bitter or pungent. There's so much variety!

These labels only point at the relative differences between energies that each of us may perceive. Of course you may prefer particular energy "flavors" over others.

Preferences are one of the great joys of living. They can, however, be used in ways that limit your willingness to explore new territories.

That said, whatever you choose, whether it is journeying into new lands or staying close to what is familiar, it is all totally fine!

There is no right or wrong way for you to move through the world. There is only what you choose and all that your choices create.

How cool is it that the world is so vast and complex that we can travel in the directions that work for each one of us in each moment? What a wild, bold adventure it is to be alive!?! Who needs TV when life itself is dramatic beyond measure?

And speaking of dramas, how many dramas are you presently starring in? Where are the people around you inventing theatrics that would put even the most imaginative screenwriters to shame? What roles have you been playing in these shows? And are they any fun for you?

What if you let go of the "rightness" and "wrongness" of everything and *enjoyed* everyone's performances? What would that be like, I wonder? Could you use your energy differently?

If you truly acknowledged and *knew* that everything is changeable, would the "problems" of your life be so daunting?

What if, rather than lamenting your life-- or the currents of energy that you encounter-- you could be present, enjoy, and dance with *everything* and be part of creating a world of joy and ease?

Are you willing to be that potent?

Why did nobody ask us these questions in high school when things got so weird!?!

Maybe, for you, these questions could have been useful even earlier than high school. Whenever it was that you were coaxed or tricked (or even forced) into moving from a playful world of exploration and curiosity into the serious world of doing the "right" things and never the "wrong" things.

What would your life be like if you'd had a companion who encouraged you to find ever greater ease and joy in the world rather than judging the seeming rightness or wrongness of your actions?

You know what? You *do* have that companion! He or she has been there with you since before you were born. It is *YOUR BODY*!!!

Yay!!!! Jackpot! Finally, someone you can hang out with who truly— pardon the pun—*HAS YOUR BACK!!*

Your body is constantly giving you a wide range of information about the world around you. What if you could use this information to your advantage?

Would you be willing to receive your own awareness and use it to create the life you most desire?

Listening to and receiving the collaborative contribution your body can be in the creation of your life might just surprise you.

Are you bold enough to try that out?

In the language of Access Consciousness®, your body is a sensory organism, primed to alert you to the shifting fields of energy through and around you.

Throughout your life you have been aware of all sorts of physical sensations. Contrary to what you might assume, not all of those sensations indicate what is occurring within *your* body or *your* life.

Yes, not all of the information that comes to you via your senses originates within you!

Just as the sounds you hear are not necessarily noises that you are making, the same is true with all sorts of other physical awareness.

We simply have not been encouraged to ask questions about what we perceive. We have, instead, been trained and rewarded to come to conclusions, or to find "answers" about everything.

And, as with judgment, we have become addicted to conclusions. Herein lies the root of "figuring things out."

How much time do you spend trying to figure things out?

What if, instead, you could approach *everything* with greater curiosity, ask more questions, and play with the information that comes your way?

What if the next time your body alerts you of something— rather than jumping to a conclusion about it—you could ask for more information?

Listening to and receiving all of the information that comes to you can assist you to make choices that are more fun for you.

Shifting your perspective and opening up to the collaborative contribution your body can be in the creation of your life might surprise you.

Let's return to my story and explore some of what is possible when you begin to work *with* the consciousness of your body.

So, I stopped riding horses. I stopped long enough to discover what their absence revealed. Navigating the strange reality of my teenage years brought up all sorts of confusion and discomfort.

Too bad the comedies and dramas on TV didn't give my being or body the joys of running, jumping, and flying through the air I'd grown so accustomed to while riding horses.

In the strangely challenging atmosphere of transitioning into the "grown up" world, I longed for the freedom of movement that being with horses encouraged.

Fortunately, my stepmother invited me to a modern dance class. Even more fortunate (and somewhat rare in the world of dance), the teacher empowered each dancer to truly be themselves as they moved through the choreography of the class.

All too often in the dance world, people are asked to mimic their teachers and choreographers. This is sold as "good technique."

It's not until reaching more advanced levels that many dancers are empowered to bring their own nuances to a dance.

I, on the other hand, was blessed with a teacher who asked us to be and express all that was within us as we moved.

She recognized that we are all incredibly unique and that the energies and qualities we bring to each movement is different for each of us.

She brought our awareness to some easy ways we can work with our bodies (such as allowing our knees to bend fluidly to absorb the impact of a jump) and encouraged us to say what WE have to say as we dance.

What a gift this teacher has been to my entire life!

Studying with her reinforced the profound joys of expressing myself with my body. And so, I danced and danced and danced.

With the blessing of my incredibly supportive parents, I threw myself into what has become a lifelong investigation of the art of embodiment.

And this is where things get super interesting!

My body has taught me about consciousness in ways that I never imagined possible.

The days I spent in the studio revealed an enormity and magnificence of physical consciousness that, even still, blows my puny little mind ALL THE TIME!

And I know that there is still more to discover.

The more I turn to my body as my ally and acknowledge its contribution to the creation of my life, the richer my life becomes. Truly, how does it get any better than that?!?!

Before I go on, though, let's stop and check in for a moment...

What is coming up for you as you read all of this?

Has your body been talking to you throughout your life?

What has it said to you? And how have you received its counsel?

Are you friendly with your body? Are you annoyed by his/her input?

Would you be willing to check in with it right now?

How comfortable are you and can you change anything to get just a little cozier?

Ok, ok, enough questions for the moment.

Let's proceed with an occasion in my life where my body woke me up to a totally different way of being.

I was in a dance class one day when I experienced a sudden, strange pain. I say strange because it came from

NOWHERE! Or, at least, that is how it seemed to me at the time. I knew that the pain I was aware of did not come from my body.

I was standing still when I noticed it and, though I no longer remember where in my body I sensed it, I knew that the sensation did not originate within me. I looked around the room and wondered where the pain came from. Who was the source of it?

It was as though, in an instant, my eyes and ears were opened and all of my senses came online! I scanned the room and was aware of the bodies and beings around me with greater clarity than before.

I recognized the staggering history of body judgment that these dancers and I had endured, and how much we were all perpetuating that same abuse on ourselves.

There I was, surrounded by incredibly talented beings staring at themselves in the mirrors, critiquing their every move. Whoa!!!

I knew that going into a dance class required courage, I just didn't realize what it was that we were encountering in the studio.

In that one moment, with that strange pain, my body gave me a world of information that changed my life forever.

I always assumed that the ways I felt about my dancing were simply areas where my technique could improve or was strong.

It never crossed my mind that I might be picking up on the thoughts, feelings, emotions, and bodies of the other dancers in the room! Who knew that was possible?!

There is a completely world changing tool in Access

Consciousness that is the simple question:

Who does this belong to?®

This leads us right back to the concept that I shared with you earlier. Who does this belong to? acknowledges the capacity that each of us has to be aware of far more beyond ourselves.

This question has been my springboard into even more questions. I am curious how far our awareness extends. And, what can we do with all that we are aware of?

Using the tool of "Who does this belong to?" allows us the space to gain more perspective on what we are encountering and opens the possibility of greater choices than we may immediately believe are available.

Let's apply this tool to something outside of the dance studio. Have you ever been sitting somewhere quietly when someone walked in who was greatly agitated or grieving or stressed out? What was that like? What did you notice? *Where* did you notice what you noticed?

Did your shoulders tense or your stomach turn? Did the quality of the room change? What impact did this person's presence have on you?

You know what it is like to get a song stuck in your head, yes?

Let's imagine that each person you encounter is singing a song. Their song plays the tune of who they are choosing to be in that moment.

They may love to sing sad, sad songs. Or grouchy songs. Or silly songs. They may use the same chords that their friends and family use. They may sing strange songs that you have never heard before. How cool is that?!

We are all walking around in a glorious, energetic symphony!

Here's a question for you: do you get other people's songs stuck in your head? Do you take on other people's energies as though you have no choice in the matter?

What would your life be like if you could listen to the songs that are being sung by the world around you without getting lost in those melodies?

How much more fun might you have if you could consciously choose what songs you are singing?

If this seems challenging, try using "who does this belong to?" Let yourself discover the immensity of your awareness!

Let yourself sing the songs that you would like to sing.

How much fun can you have singing such different sounds (or energies) that your voice changes the tune of the world?

What would it be like to walk through the world with a presence that changes everything and everyone you come in contact with?

Would you be willing to show up and contribute to the symphony?

Will you allow your awareness and presence to encourage, tickle, and enchant the world around you?

A dance teacher of mine used to tell me about a dream of hers: to stand on stage alone and do nothing but slowly look from one side of the audience to the other.

She wondered what it would take for her performance to be so clear, so strong that the audience be riveted.

135

She was, without a doubt, someone who could speak volumes with a single glance-- like an upset mother quieting her rowdy kids with the slight raise of an eyebrow.

This image of a simple, almost motionless performance captivates me.

What is it that we see when we look at that woman on the stage? She is performing for us, responding to us as she leads our gaze.

Wow! The vulnerability required to be scrutinized, willing to truly be seen-- even demanding it—necessitates enormous potency.

This illusive quality that so many performers seek to cultivate, *this is PRESENCE*!

Whether we acknowledge it or not, presence is an aspect of our very being, an innate gift. What we choose to do and to create with our presence is entirely up to us; the possibilities are limitless!

I wonder... what will you choose now? Are you courageous enough to set down your judgments and your conclusions?

Do you dare to let your awareness be sharp and clear as you move through the chaotic energies you encounter?

And, will you allow your body to assist you in the creation and enjoyment of your reality?

These days I take greater pleasure in the world around me. Now that my senses are open in ways they were not when I was younger, I take part in the many unfolding dramas I perceive with a delight I never dreamed possible.

I was walking through the French Quarter in New Orleans the other day. The weather was glorious! The air was cool. The sun was shining. The tourists were excited. And it smelled delicious!

For two blocks, I was immersed in what I can best describe as a grand sensory sculpture. The environment was thick with a smorgasbord of varied energies that were mouth watering.

Everywhere I turned I was hit with a different, rich and inviting sensation. For a moment I felt as though I were a master chef, aware of a million distinct, exquisite flavors. I was suddenly so hungry that I wanted to eat EVERYTHING!

A couple passed by and I sensed their story. He emanated a desire to be recognized as capable and important with a strong undercurrent of wanting to please his female companion.

She shone with the delight of being taken care of, accented by a shadow of cold dissatisfaction. The quality of their relationship was complex and specific and full of history and... it passed by me in an instant!

It washed over me like the tantalizing scents in the Louisiana air. I drank it in. My hunger subsided as I enjoyed all of the subtle nuances I perceived in that space: a full range of energies from intense and somewhat rotten to delicate, tender, and refreshing.

If I knew every word in every language on Earth, I would still be hard pressed to describe all that my body and being senses. What I can say is that it is wild and magnificent and constantly inspiring me to move!

What about you? What are you aware of?

What contribution are you to this glorious universe that is bursting forth through and around us?

Will you join me in the joyful creation of a world that

exceeds all expectations?

Oh please, oh please, will you dance with me?

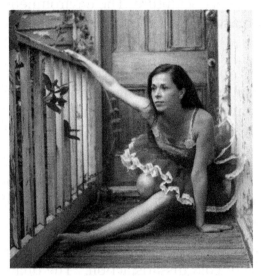

Photo by: Bobby Bonsey

Monica Mata Gilliam

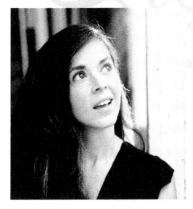

Monica Mata Gilliam is a Dancer, Acupuncturist, Author, Access Consciousness® Certified Facilitator, and Talk to the Entities™ Certified Facilitator. She is committed to joyfully expanding the possibilities of conscious embodiment.

Monica received a Bachelor of Arts in Dance from Texas Woman's University. After performing and creating in the Pacific Northwest, she suffered an injury leading her to visit an acupuncturist for treatment. Curious, she explored the world of energy with Traditional Chinese Medicine.

She received a Masters of Acupuncture and Oriental Medicine from the Seattle Institute of Oriental Medicine and set out to contribute to the bodies and beings of this world. One day she stumbled across Access Consciousness and her world exploded into infinite sparkling possibilities!

Monica encourages people to step into the lives and bodies they most desire through facilitation, bodywork, and life-changing movement and consciousness classes.

Her schedule, adventures, and eager contribution can be found by visiting her website:

www.MonicaMataGilliam.com

Chapter 8

That Ecstatic Moment
by Katherine McIntosh CFMW

We dance for *laughter,* We dance for *tears,*

We dance for *madness,* We dance for *fears,*

We dance for *hopes,* We dance for *screams,*

We are the *dancers.* We create *dreams.*

Have you ever had a time in your life where your entire body and being buzz with the ecstatic energy of aliveness?

Some people experience this when they are falling in love, in the act of a really good romp in the hay, some when they are participating in sports, or even watching sports, and some when they do something they've never done before.

It's that ecstatic moment when every cell in your body

buzzes with the aliveness of being and you forget everything in your life.

Nothing exists except for that moment...you are alive, aware, awake, and the joy of the moment envelops your entire being. It's like a complete adrenaline rush of possibilities. Sweat pouring off every inch of your body, and the smile of internal ecstasy takes you to the edges of the universe and back.

Everything seems possible. The rush of beauty pumps in every cell of your being.... you are beautiful and you remember what the aliveness of being is all about.

For me, dance and movement create this sense of dynamic creation where the body and being align with the infinite possibilities of the universe.... where anything and everything seems possible.

There are few things in this life that I have found that bring me to the kinesthetic memory of that aliveness of being more than dance.

Dance creates communion, connection, release, and renewal.

There is this intimate experience and connection that gets created when you give the body permission to move in its own way...absent of judgment, absent of shoulds and shouldn'ts, absent of the past... it brings you to the present moment of truly discovering what the body is possible of creating. And when you awake to the present moment, your vision gets clearer, old memories get released, and the space of the NOW envelops you.

I dance because there's no greater feeling in the world than moving to a piece of music and letting the rest of the world disappear.

And there certainly is magic in that moment where no one and nothing else exists besides you and the moment of being entirely with your body.

It doesn't matter what you find in your life, but when you find it, you know it is something that contributes an aliveness of being and body that can't be found anywhere else.

For me that moment was dance. It found me when I most needed it in my life. I was broken down, sick, exhausted, over-worked, under-nourished, on the brink of despair, depression, disease, and an overall disdain for life. Dance revived me and revived my life.

Movement has always been a passion of mine, but I never thought I'd be a dancer. I was a soccer player, a volleyball player, a downhill skier, hiker, mountain biker, runner.... but dancer... not a chance!

And then, I went to college. I was over 1500 miles away from home. I was struggling with my self-esteem, body weight, and image. I had no idea who I was or what I was supposed to be. I was supposed to know what I wanted to be when I grew up and honestly I had no clue. So I signed up for a modern dance class.

There was a moment when I was asked to lead the entire class... I thought... who me?

I've never danced in my life and you want me to lead the class!

It was the longest, scariest 5 minutes of my life....and yet.....something in those 5 minutes broke open in a way I just can't explain.

The entire class was smiling, moving, waving, shouting, ecstatic. The teacher came up to me after and said, she'd never seen someone engage the entire class...she looked at me and said I had something special.

I had heard that same thing from my coaches "I was special"... "I had something" ... In an environment that was completely foreign to me, in a physical setting where I felt the most out of place... it was the beginning of me being willing to take risks and go outside of my comfort zone. It was the beginning of me falling in love with dance.

If my body could take me on the adventure of living in a totally different way, then what else was I capable of doing?

And so began an adult love affair with movement and dance. Without me knowing it, movement became my medicine. I had taken a break from it, slightly abandoned it, but never truly forgotten about it.

At the age of 26, I was brought to my knees by a health condition that no one and nothing was able to solve. I was depressed, desolate, and practically dying. I was falling apart. Dance and movement found their way back into my life when I most needed them. They helped me heal.

You see, movement of any kind literally opens up your body's ability to heal. When we repeat the same movement over and over again, whether it is a destructive movement or a generative movement, then we allow the body to establish patterns according to the movement.

If your movement is to constantly be worried about your life, your body, your health, or your aging, then you will establish deeper patterns of the same "movement" therefore increasing pain, struggle, worry, etc. However, if your movement is catered toward generative momentum, then you can shift.

Whenever I feel stuck in my life, I move my body.

I go for a run, get on my mountain bike, or play music in my house. I move my body. However you desire to move your body, just MOVE it... each movement allows for a different possibility to show up. Movement is also the willingness to stay and be in the question with your body. One of the biggest things that shifted my health when 9 months of doctor visits, scans, tests, MRIs, and evaluations couldn't solve it, was the willingness to be curious with my body.

The doctors were always guessing and then prescribing me medication based on the diagnosis...well that never solved it because, truth be told, it never addressed the underlying issues causing the symptoms in the first place.

Healing is the by-product of consciousness.

If you are willing to BE the question, then the body can re-organize itself.

If you continue to deliver conclusions, and half-ass attempts at answers that you think will solve it, then the body maintains the disease. I remember at some point in my health journey, I realized that the doctor's were guessing as much as I was...and truth be told they had no idea!

When I realized this, I took matters into my own hands. I was introduced to a woman (through dance) who offered the possibility that she might be able to help my body.

She didn't have any pre-conceived notions of what was wrong, she just knew that something was wrong. Until we connected to my body and being, went underneath the surface, then we wouldn't truly ever know what was causing the disease in the first place.

In a one-hour session 50% of my symptoms had completely disappeared. That one session changed more than what 9 months of doctors, therapists, medicine and tests failed to.

That one hour was an exploration about what my body knew.

It was then that I was able to see everything that was actually true. I was living a lie. I had to start to open my eyes and truly take a look at everything I had created. It was like the experience of being an eagle flying over head, looking at my life from an observing witness that had no point of view.

From that perspective, I was able to look at the things in my life and the truth about my choices that I didn't want to see.

So often, we avoid the things we don't want to see for fear of what or who we might lose. What I've discovered is that when we are willing to acknowledge where we are and what we create by our choices, then everything has a chance to change.

That one hour gave me a burst of energy and space and ease that I had been missing for a long time. That's when I knew that this experience was opening me up to a whole new possibility I hadn't even considered. From that point forward I began to be curious about my body, ask it questions, be an open invitation and move with it from the question, not from the demand of telling it how it should move. It wasn't about getting my body "in" a position, it was about asking...

- **Body, how do you want to move?**

- **What do you want to show me?**

- **What would be fun for you?**

When I finally invited my body to show me how it wanted to dance and move, my entire life of anger, sadness, pain, rage, abuse, and repressed emotions began to release. The more I danced the happier I got. The clearer I got. And the more I began to trust myself in a way I was never willing to do before.

Those moments changed my life.

I didn't have to spend 2 hours a week sitting on a couch in a stale room with a stiff therapist spouting advice at me. Instead, I'd put on comfy clothes and dance barefoot to music. Music that moved me, inspired me, coerced me, invited me. It was cathartic and I felt alive. The dance allowed me to connect to EVERYTHING in my life; the good, the bad, the ugly, the beautiful.

Dance taught me that nothing is permanent. Life is constantly changing.

Dance can be a metaphor for life. It too is constantly changing. Movement taught me that if I can move through an intense moment or emotion or trauma in the dance, I can also move through it in my life.

The body stores memories. And, when we invite the body to move, it can release these hidden memories. Every new movement we create with the body allows something new to open up.

When you allow your body to be and live and move as the question, then you can find movements that can heal and release trauma, abuse, pain, feelings of lack and low self-worth. In that same movement you can also open up new neural pathways and create new patterns and behaviors.

You see. I spent over 10 years and over $100,000 on therapy. Every week I'd go to the therapist and I would talk. I'd process left, right, and center and I'd walk out of there a little lighter. I'd have a game plan. "This week would be different," I'd think to myself. And then life would happen and I'd find myself in a similar wounded hole just like the week before. Different story, same game...something was wrong with me and if I only had enough will power or more determination, or I was willing to meditate or practice my way out of my triggered states of behavior, then I'd be okay.

But the problem with that train of thought is you cannot use your cognitive mind to get you out of unconscious behaviors that are hidden underneath the surface.

Most trauma and drama lives in the reptilian brain...the one focused solely on survival. It's this reptilian brain that is responsible for fight or flight....It has one thing it cares about: survival.

So when it gets signaled, it sends an instantaneous knee jerk reaction to your survival skills. And when that happens, no amount of cognitive talk therapy (engaging the logical brain) has been able to get to the root of what's causing the behavior in the first place.

It's not the behavior that's the problem, it's what's underneath the surface. I don't know about you, but using my limited mind to talk me out of my biggest emotional triggers only gets me more stuck, more confused, more depressed, and more convinced that something must be wrong with me!

Change is almost always never cognitive.

My solution: Dance it out!

When we engage the body to contribute to the possibilities that the mind can't see, there is this alchemical creation that begins to open up. It's like an internal fire that releases old patterns, habits, thoughts, feelings, and emotions that we didn't even know were there.

For me, no amount of processing truly changed the underlying behavior. But creating a new movement and committing to dancing it out instead of resisting it allowed stuck patterns in my life to change and heal with total ease. It was quick, painless, and euphoric. And it engaged my body in a new memory that lasted way longer than trying to talk my way into a new behavior.

My body got happier and the things in my personal life that I had been hiding from or pretending were okay started to get really clear.

What I first had to look at was that at 25 years old, I decided to marry the first man I fell in love with. I was naïve, young, and, truth be told, I didn't believe enough in myself to think that anyone would love me.

So when this dark skinned Latin man from South America started to notice me, I dove head first into a very torrid love affair. I ignored a lot of red flags and warning signs.

At the time, I thought, if we loved each other enough, we could get through anything. Boy was I wrong!

Looking back at that time in my life, I laugh. Lucky for me, I have an incredible ability to find the humor and gift of my choices instead of seeing any of my choices as a problem. (You would think that when he didn't speak ANY English, I would have been willing to run in the other direction)

"If you can't get rid of the skeleton in your closet, you'd best teach it to dance."
~George Bernard Shaw

It was during this wake up call, that dance brought me back to life. I danced everyday. In fact, I fell in love with it so much, I got certified to facilitate women (and men) of all walks of life to dance, move their bodies, be in the question, and pay attention to that moment where everything disappears and it's just you, your body, and the moment.

I taught dance and movement for over 15 years. It was those moments and memories that allowed me to be present with the incredible gift our bodies are. I watched women and men who never thought they could dance fall in love with dance and in turn fall in love with themselves.

There is something inexplicable that happens when the

As long as you're dancing, you can break the rules.

— *Mary Oliver* —

body trusts itself to move.

When you invite the body
to be the question and contribute,
new neural pathways will open the door
to a whole new way of being.

I wonder what you know about movement and how your body likes to move?

I've always been a rule breaker. Bodies don't follow rules. They follow possibilities. If you're following the rules, chances are you're not totally listening to your body.

It doesn't matter if you don't dance. What matters is that you break the rules and listen to your body instead of listening to the rules that you've been told about bodies.

No one can tell you more about you and your body than you. Nobody knows more about you and your body than you.

So wake up and find your own dance. This journey is meant to be fun! Enjoy the music....it might just be inviting you to a whole new possibility with your body to wake up to your life and actually find your way into joy.

I remember my first dance class in college. I felt so out of place. A soccer player and down hill skier was taking a modern dance class?

I felt awkward and unsure of myself and it wasn't until my teacher invited me to lead the class that I realized I had the power to help people find their joy.

I also remember being completely surprised by the idea that my teacher saw in me...a dancer.

Great dancers are defined by the physical connection they have to their bodies, the music, the moment, the emotion, and everything in between.

I remember my first ever solo performance was in grad school and I performed in front of over 200 people.... I remember being so NERVOUS! I had never performed before...not like that...and it was a solo act.

I was nervous, sick, and exhausted. There was that moment right before going on stage where I thought to myself... I don't know if I can do this.... and then I thought...What have I got to lose?

The director came up to me afterwards and said that he had spent 30 years directing & teaching dance and that I might not have been the most technically perfect, but the sensations the audience left with were palpable.

He said he wished every single dancer could emote through their bodies the way I did. In that moment I knew it wasn't about getting it perfect, but more about moving whatever it is I felt or needed to express.

So often when we get stuck, we want to process, talk about it, journal about it, understand it, try and change it. Well honestly, one of the quickest ways I've discovered to change it, is to move your body...shake it out...release it out of the cells...then it can change.

It's in breaking out of our comfort zone and trusting our bodies in a whole new way that life and the magic of life, in all its possibilities, can show you a whole new way.

When you function and move with your body as a question, then your body will play with you, invite you, communicate with you, and connect with you.

This dance, this journey called life, it's about that connection. It's about trusting you anywhere at anytime and it's about inviting the body to dance with you.

Whatever your dance is, find it, trust it, move with it, and invite it to show you all the possibilities you didn't even know were possible.

Katherine McIntosh

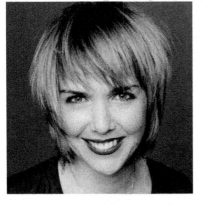

Katherine McIntosh is an International speaker and facilitator on the topics of health, wealth, business, body, consciousness, and living a vibrant lifestyle. She is an Intuitive Consultant & Body Expert who combines the wisdom of the body with the possibilities for business and personal expansion. She has helped thousands of people change the things they think they cannot change.

She is the founder of the No Judgment Diet, an International course in possibilities for the body that has helped hundreds of people in over 18 different countries get out of judgment with their bodies and create the business and life they love!

She is passionate about helping women and men connect to the wisdom of the body. Katherine is an expert working with the energies and systems of the body to change the entire blueprint of someone's life. Katherine treats each person from the perspective that their situation is unique.

For more information, please visit:

www.katherinemcintosh.com

www.nojudgmentdiet.com

The End

SECRET BONUSES JUST FOR YOU!

Require more information?
Desire more for you and for your body?
Got questions?

Check out our *Secret Bonuses Membership* site.

To access the site for free go to:

dancingasthebodyofconsciousness.com/secretbonuses

and enter your email address.

What if this is just the beginning? The beginning of a new adventure discovering the magic within your body and the ways he/she can contribute to your life and living?

We would love to invite you to this new possibility!

We've created a place with additional resources, inspirational videos, quotes and much more so that you may begin your journey today.

These resources will guide you in having more joy, awareness, communion and fun with your body.

How much fun can you have with your body now?

Enjoy and thank you again for purchasing *Dancing as the Body of Consciousness!*

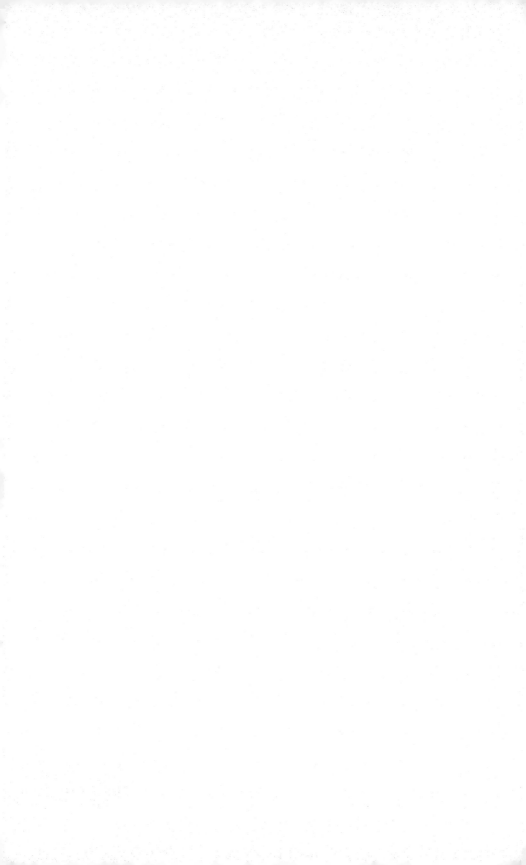

Lightning Source UK Ltd.
Milton Keynes UK
UKOW05f2323230517
301881UK00001B/96/P